The Secret Gift

What They Don't Want You to Know About Lyme Disease

Excerpts from the Journal
"The Chronicles of Despair"

Stephen E. Amsden

South Berkshire Press

ISBN 978-1-60166-049-7

DISCLAIMER: The contents of this book are intended for informational and educational purposes only and not for the purpose of rendering medical advice. This book is not intended to be a substitute for professional medical advice, diagnosis, or treatment. Always seek the advice of your physician or other qualified health provider (ideally a Lyme-Literate Medical Doctor) with any questions you may have regarding any existing or suspected medical condition.

CONTENTS

DEDICATIONS & ACKNOWLEDGEMENTS

This work is dedicated to my mother, Jean Currier Amsden, who gave me life twice; once when I was born, and again at age forty-nine when she demanded I get a third Lyme test at IGeneX; to my father Henry H. Amsden for his gentle kindness and caring hand in guiding me in a life of inner contemplation; and to two LLMD (Lyme literate medical doctors) who shall remain anonymous for their dedication and willingness to get me to the finish line; to Marcy Lackey, Angel of Light, Caretaker during my recovery; to Pam Harrison for her continued love, support and companionship in the aftermath; and to my beloved Newfoundland "Kelsey" for dragging me on to the finish line—and beyond.

PREFACE TO THE FIRST EDITION

This story is unlike any other. Testimony to triumph over not just Lyme disease, but of conquering fear and denial by overcoming the source of human suffering. Beyond frequently cited causes and purported failures in treatment, long-term antibiotic therapy remains our best advantage against the Borrelia spirochete.

Contrary to popular belief, Lyme disease is easy to get and hard to cure, not the other way around. And yes, it can display a rash, but not in most cases. There is no 100% accurate test for the disease, and it is frequently missed by standard blood tests. It is found in every state and on every continent other than Antarctica, not just the northeast United States. There is growing evidence that it can be transmitted sexually, from expectant mother to unborn fetus, and remains undetected in a portion of the public blood supply and in donated organs from infected people.

Alarmingly there is a new generation being born with Lyme disease by unsuspecting young mothers who themselves are unknowingly infected. Lyme disease is often misdiagnosed as one or more of the many chronic illnesses by "specialists" who deny the disease exists. The long-held myth as the "Great Imitator" of modern chronic illnesses is slowly yielding to evidence as the "Great Originator" of severe mental and physical impairment. Consequences are debilitating, and can be fatal if not identified and treated properly. Too often people who remain undiagnosed are at a far greater risk of violent behavior or suicide.

Long-term antibiotic treatment still remains the best option for treatment.

Depending on the length and severity of the infection, it can take months or perhaps years for the disease to subside. Nearly all those who undertake antibiotic treatment, *long-term*, see real improvement in quality of life and a higher probability of *cure*.

The Modern Dilemma of Human Suffering

Often in the darkness before dawn is revealed our greatest gifts. Our experience in these times, as all previous generations have encountered, trials and tribulations will continue to test the veracity, patience and understanding as will generations to come. The silent epidemic of Lyme disease is not unlike the plagues described in the history books, perhaps for one difference – could it be that this current plague is a modified creature born of science, man-made, and not a creature of nature itself? Is the current Lyme spirochete the first Genetically Modified Organism (GMO), a creature of mankind's diabolical impulse for self-destruction? Or is it possible that *all* plagues and diseases are man-made? As incredulous as this sounds, the question is poignant in the larger picture, for mankind is both part of nature and part of something else, and subject to mysteries that transcend here and now. This journey leads beyond Lyme disease, a story of overcoming incredible odds, of redemption and salvation.

This timeless journey transcends everyday existence in the attempt to answer the elusive questions of our best philosophical inquiries which have generated more questions than answers. Embracing the difficult question of "why" this peculiar conspiracy of silence surrounds the perplexing ordeal of Lyme disease is a spiritual journey of transformation and re-generation of the human spirit.

Recognizing the source of human affliction itself, not just Lyme disease but the source of all human suffering and misery, requires acknowledging lessons both past, present and future. Current manifestations of Lyme, as in all disease, are inherently afflictions of the human spirit. Whether suffering is to be cured or endured remains one of the ultimate paradoxes of human existence, and ultimately a personal choice. That history repeats itself endlessly is undeniable evidence of this.

Herein lies the ultimate source of our suffering, and specifically its role in us, and our role in it.

PART 1:

A Brief History of Misdiagnosis Over 34 Years

The narrative of this journey began in 1977 in a series of personal journals kept for over thirty years, aptly entitled "*The Chronicles of Despair.*" Within it are described the anguish and turmoil of battling against an unknown illness from age fifteen to its discovery at age forty-nine. Revealed in this narrative are the underlying forces at work that apply to every single individual human being, and not just those afflicted by Lyme disease. Particular emphasis is dedicated to all of those on their path to awareness and self-discovery while overcoming the obstacles that inevitably rise up as the many challenges we face on our way "home." Let's face this journey together and know that we are not alone.

1974: First Misdiagnosis—EPILEPSY

Since the mid-1960's, my memory of the vacations I took nearly every summer since I was eight years old in Brewster, Massachusetts on Cape Cod, right in the crook of the arm, bay side, were comprised of sunsets over the water and the tide way out over the sandbars, baking in the sun. My parents, aunts and uncles, and grandparents would all schedule the much-anticipated rendezvous at the Cape, usually during the weeks of February in sharp contrast to the harsh and dreary winters so characteristic of New Hampshire. These excursions to the beach sometimes stretched out beyond Hyannis Port to the long-protected dunes of Truro, and further out to the tip of Provincetown. Not far inland from Brewster is the renowned Nickerson's State Park, known for its tall whispering pines, roses, rabbits and deer. Some evenings the whole family would pile into a couple of station wagons and go searching for rabbits, the most sightings claiming victory. As active youngsters, with my younger brother Nathan, we would explore the marshes and inlets along the breakwaters sporting the long, tall grass that could cut if you were not careful.

Several years later in 1974, now at fifteen years old, it was the teenage girls from Brockton, Massachusetts that had my attention, mostly on the beach. But sometimes this would turn into walks along the inlets, through the tall grass and the stubborn brine drenched sod that held it together through the ebb and flow of the tides. There, and numerous times at home as in central-southern small towns all throughout New England, it was not unusual to find an occasional tick on us, which was no real cause for alarm. After all, let's face it—we were outdoor kids and lovers of nature. Nothing could keep us out of the woods. It was during these early years I began noticing small, split second flashes of light that would interrupt my thought process. Like small erratic firings of electrical charges, these were not so bothersome as to affect my otherwise "normal" development, and nothing was mentioned about them. It did not occur to me at the time to be something abnormal. Often these would be triggered by flashing lights, mostly from the sun behind the trees while passing by them while riding in the car. An ever so brief trembling or random nearly imperceptible states of split-second unconsciousness was accepted as just a normal part of growing up.

We returned home to Weare, New Hampshire in mid-July to find a garden choked with weeds. The family all agreed to tackle it together and set about the task. Hot day, humid, in the 90's, sweat running down the face, I bent down pulling on ragweed, and stopped for an instant, stood up, and whoa—the blood went right to my head. Dizzy.... blinking my eyes, everything turned silvery, fuzzy as I steadied my steps along the path. And there, under the large maple tree at the head of the garden on the east side, appeared a shimmering, undulating globe of multi-colored lights, a pink cloud about the size of a beachball about three-feet wide. It shone with the brilliance of a small sun, emanating power and overwhelming energy. As if in the presence of a higher intelligence, an angel, or vision, I was overcome with an intense feeling of awe. Shining with a brilliant iridescence and intense beauty that defies description, all of the colors of the rainbow changing and undulating within it. I pointed and exclaimed to the rest of my family "Look!" As it floated across the yard, driveway, above the car and up and over the roof of the house and disappeared, I fell back being rendered completely unconscious by the experience.

Coming back to consciousness after several minutes on the ground, I am looking straight into the family dog's face, who was checking out what just happened with great interest and concern. Several days later, we are on to Concord Hospital for the inevitable tests. Blood, EEG, and spinal tap revealed nothing. The doctors noted short, split second jolts or interruptions in concentration when looking at flashing lights during the EEG, and with that came the first misdiagnosis; *epilepsy*. The doctor advised refraining from ladders and swimming, and that it would take a year without any other seizures before I could apply for my driver's permit. This came as a shock, as it would for any teenager anticipating the newfound freedom that comes with a driver's license. We came home with a towering bottle of pills—Dilantin, three times per day, 90 pills for one month—with twelve refills. It stood ominously and looked conspicuous in the middle of the kitchen table, a tower of testament to the great power of pharmacopoeia. How little I knew then what was to come in the presence of this ominous omen.

1984: Second Misdiagnosis—MILD DEPRESSION/ANXIETY

Stubborn pride and vanity about one's health is the first stumbling block to well-being. After three years at the University of Hartford came marriage and our first daughter, Natalie, was born in 1981. Work for a local surveyor, which combined the skills obtained while working in my father's business during the 1970's with my studies at the university, sustained us, but the call to come work for NASA at the Goddard Space Flight Center in Greenbelt, Maryland in software testing was like a dream come true. As a child, dreams of becoming an astronaut and the first person to go to Mars made the decision an obvious choice, and we were Maryland-bound. At first, the work at Goddard was terrifying, as it would to someone such as myself, being inexperienced. But I soon acclimated and adapted to a new way of life, with all rewards that come from courage and perseverance in a new career.

With the misdiagnosis of epilepsy ten years earlier long forgotten and a thing of the past, there was nothing but a bright and exciting future that lay ahead. There was no recurrence of the Gran-Mal seizure that had struck in 1975, which had been attributed to a "fluke" in the wake of growing and developing as a teenager into adulthood. After the one-year sentence of no swimming, no climbing and a postponed driver's license, back then at age seventeen I was considered in all respects an otherwise completely normal and thriving adolescent. However, ten years later in

1984, at age 25, the brief occurrences of unconsciousness due to "flashing lights" were ever present, but still ignored. New interests in music spawned a parallel life in the evenings and nights after work, and often it would be 1:00am before turning in for five hours of sleep before putting on the suit and tie the next morning in preparation for another day's work in the real world at Goddard.

Normal pressures of being a young working father, husband and part-time musician were relished challenges, and an underlying disturbance or low form of anxiety seemed normal given the responsibilities for anyone in similar circumstances. Yet, the pressure tipped the balance into a frenzied, almost imperceptible feeling that emerged as an obstacle to everyday life and became increasingly intolerable. The feeling, though not overwhelming at the time, began to interfere in gradual increments and became more difficult to overcome. Ambition exacts its price and takes its toll, and I reassured myself that this was the price for it, as there was always so much left to be done and limited hours in a day. Doggedly, I kept up the pace, and the family doctor referred me to a specialist who prescribed Librium (the original chlordiazepoxide HCI and prototype for the benzodiazepine compounds) for mild depression and anxiety. This alleviated the symptoms but also the drive to succeed in the music business, as it interrupted the creative flow of writing and performing music. The interference with this creative impulse was simply unacceptable at the time, and the course of medication was immediately and abruptly discontinued.

1990: Third Misdiagnosis—MANIC DEPRESSION

The incident in 1984, when prescribed Librium for mild anxiety/depression, was no big deal. Life has bumps in the road for everyone. The next six years exuded all the virtues of youth and good health: robustness, ambition, and restlessness, but with an uneasy feeling that underneath the surface something was deeply wrong. Career advancement, moving to a new home, and a new car were normal activities during the mid-1980's. But something I could not quite put my finger on, some type of background interference, a feeling that I was running out of time persisted...

The next twenty-plus years, through 1996, sees the slow but steady progression of the affliction and the gradual development of neuro-psychosis. During this time, life was focused on those things that matter most to anyone maturing into adulthood. Graduating high school, going on to college, marriage, and children, all gave plenty of motive for accomplishment, success and realizing our dreams. And we did. In 1987, then 28 years of age and in the full prime of life, now a software test engineer at the NASA Goddard Space Flight Center in Greenbelt, Maryland doing systems integration for satellite imaging and FAA traffic systems, the sensation of numbness in both forearms just before sleep did not bother me much. But in my parallel life as a music recording producer, excessive "burnout" from a compilation LP recording venture revealed signs of stress. After listening to and reviewing the first 900 recordings submitted for the project, there was an inkling of something amiss. Soon unable to overcome reluctance to continue with the project, I began procrastinating. With imminent contractual deadlines just around the corner, it seemed odd that I could no longer continue to be effective.

Attributing it to life itself was easy. Living two parallel lives—the daytime job at NASA and rock musician at night—in 1988 I decided to assign a share of the load to the vice president of our indie label, *Empire Records International*, and relocate with my family back to New Hampshire, where I took up working once again for my father in land surveying. My brothers and I had worked in the family business on and off during summers and weekends as teens, and into adulthood as well. Business was booming in the late 1980's and afforded almost daily trips into the woods. We were used to it, and took the extremes of heat and cold, insects, and poison ivy all as part of the game. Ticks were found occasionally and treated topically to "prevent infection."

The everyday pressures as a business manager brought with it the typical challenges and successes that one might expect. But just two years into this new challenge the economy was descending into a severe recession that began to threaten our very livelihood. The drop off in work necessitated layoffs in a dramatically short period of time. At our passive-solar home in Epsom, I recall standing in the forest near the house and looking out over the valley to the mountain off in the distance and experiencing the most pervasive feeling of dread, as if standing on the edge of an abyss yawning before me. It was easy to attribute this metaphor to the dwindling economy, yet something about it seemed all-the-more imminent. The alternating experience of exhilaration with private life and the lows of the working world led the family doctor this time to prescribe yet another course of anti-depressants for manic depression; this time,

Lithium. This worked well in alleviating the worse parts of the lows but left a residual feeling of being "stuck in a hole." The side effects of treatment eventually wore out its welcome, being worse than the symptoms, and treatment was discontinued after just a few months.

1996: Fourth Misdiagnosis—BI-POLAR DEPRESSION

Attending a series of concerts during the summer of 1995 brought on a nagging sore throat that wouldn't go away for three months. No visible sign of irritation, no strep, but it hurt bad. After two 30-day rounds of different antibiotics with no success, on the phone the doc explained he would call a specialist he knew and ask his opinion. After waiting anxiously by the phone, the recommendation was for one more course of antibiotics—this time, Erythromycin (an antibiotic for the treatment of a number of bacterial infections, including respiratory tract infections, skin infections, chlamydia infections, and syphilis.) His colleague thought it might be something called "mycoplasma." Within hours of beginning the new regimen, the sore throat was finally draining away.

However, not long after in 1996, upon purchasing a new home, the pressure seemed overwhelming, and a new job brought with it an onerous feeling of extreme dread. At the family doctor's office this time the diagnosis was yet again depression: *bi-polar depression*, and I was prescribed Serzone (Nefazodone), an SSRI anti-depressant. (Serotonin-specific reuptake inhibitors are a class of drugs that are typically used as antidepressants in the treatment of major depressive disorder and anxiety disorders.) That seemed to do the trick. It worked well, and I continued with it for the next seven years. These were the most productive years of my life.

Bigger responsibilities and staying ahead of bills had their priorities. Purchasing a piece of land on the beautiful Blackwater River, by the old family camp, and building our dream home, amongst other real estate ventures, musical endeavors, career and business choices, all made for huge sacrifices in time, energy and eventually, abilities. Then again emerged a creeping and increasingly pervasive form of *anxiety*. The feelings of dread returned with a vengeance, bringing a distortion of time and tremendous pressure that had me questioning my ability to continue. This time I was referred to a psychiatrist. I couldn't believe it. What the *hell* is going on? What is *wrong* with me? But at that time there was still faith and trust in the health-care system, and I never doubted that a doctor would always act in the best interest of the patient. It wasn't until much later that it became self-evident that this is not always the case. No attempt was ever made or even considered *to find an actual cause*, and this pattern of exclusion of diagnosis in favor of only treating symptoms was repeated, yet again as it had in the past.

1999: Fifth Misdiagnosis—CHRONIC ANXIETY DISORDER (PTSD)

In the late 1990's, new symptoms of severe panic, anxiety and inability to concentrate manifested as a permanent condition similar to Post Traumatic Stress Disorder (PTSD), and previous symptoms of depression got worse. These symptoms brought on more doctors, and with those, more prescriptions. Growing issues with concentration and focus increased the dosages. Panic attacks were treated with Benzodiazepines. (Benzodiazepines generally share the same pharmacological properties, such as anxiolytic, sedative, hypnotic, skeletal muscle relaxant, amnesic and anticonvulsants). Treatment first started at low doses of Lorazepam, which were gradually increased, and eventually substituted for the stronger Clonazepam, also in gradually increasing dosages. These were eventually increased over ten-fold. Eventually, I began taking the equivalent of over 100 Valium per day, and it still wasn't enough. Lamictal, Risperdal, Lithium, Prozac and more were added. My psychiatrist basically ran out of drugs to prescribe. The FDA could not approve enough new drugs fast enough to keep up with my ever-increasing symptoms.

Soon the "toxic cocktail" itself rivaled the malady. The out-of-control roller coaster was just beginning, and I was squarely stuck on the slippery slope of a pharmacology experiment gone astray as my chorus of doctors said in unison, "*It's all in your head.*"

Little did any of us know at the time how true that statement was, but not in the context it was made.

The psychiatrists were doing their best, or so it was believed at the time. Tit for tat, action-reaction based analysis, followed up with a blend of chemicals that would suppress the worst of the symptoms. Basically, "whack-a-mole" therapy. No doctor ever tried to search for the actual source of the problem, or even asked more than superficial questions about why this might be happening. Still, I doggedly did as told, believing in the underlying principle of "first do no harm."

Psychiatry continued to provide what it does best: administer drugs to alleviate and compensate for the worst of the symptoms. The attempt was never to cure, but to make the existing condition tolerable.

"We can't (or won't) identify or fix the underlying problem, but we can make you feel a lot better about it,"

...seemed to be the consistent answer. Their job was not to identify the source of the problem, but neither was it for all the other so-called "specialists" seen over the years. No one took responsibility for that. Each specialist had their own narrow view, and their own slice of the pie. Adding a psychologist did not help. They too took the side of:

"What is wrong is the way you're looking at the things."

The message seemed to be:

"Everything appears to be okay, you just have to see it the right way. It's all about your attitude."

Living with this dialogue for many years took its toll. Self-esteem dropped. Purpose, identity—all were being systematically destroyed, and no one would even make the attempt to find out why.

2001: Sixth Misdiagnosis—ATTENTION DEFICIT DISORDER (ADD)

As network administrator of the Merrimack Valley School District during year 2000, there came increasingly difficult challenges in managing multiple school locations and the many networks and computers required to run the district's technology program. These challenges involved analysis and resolution of complicated network and operating systems problems, which was my specialty of expertise. At the time I was also juggling a consulting business begun in 1996 called *Interact–Advanced System Technologies*. It was paying off, with multiple contracts with other school districts and local businesses, but it also furnished a steady stream of financial and personal pressure. It was no surprise that two years earlier the misdiagnosis of chronic anxiety disorder was arrived at.

Ever more noticeably and with increasing frequency came this creeping inability to maintain focus. This was easily attributed to the increasing load of responsibilities that came with success from our various enterprises, but the crippling effects were becoming all-the-more noticeable. Now also a landlord, with real estate investments in multi-family homes and apartment buildings, the trials and tribulations that come with having tenants were also inherited. Maintenance and evictions were frequent visitors to the high stress world already manifest, and it became increasingly evident these brought with them inherent difficulties with concentration.

All these accumulating symptoms were easily justified by these external circumstances. Steady appointments and trips to the psychiatrist and the psychologist for worsening symptoms brought its own share of additional prescriptions. Under the circumstances, it was not difficult for my doctor to pronounce Attention Deficit Disorder (ADD) as the latest additional misdiagnosis. As a result, Adderall was added to the pile of prescription bottles that littered the kitchen counter.

2003: Seventh Misdiagnosis—CARDITIS

Then, on a trip to Maryland in 2003, I suddenly found myself in the emergency room with heart arrhythmias. Three days of testing showed no signs of a heart attack, but a "dark shadow" appeared in the tissue of the heart on one of the x-rays. The attending physician finally let me go, but only reluctantly after a long, hard penetrating look of concern. There was one thing for certain—there was something very wrong here, and I could no longer hold back the creeping doubt in the back of my mind that the elephant in the room was being deliberately ignored.

Earlier in the spring of that year, a previous sensation occurred; a disturbance in the area of the heart, like a "shifting" feeling that was difficult to describe. I felt as if there had been some type of "movement" as if something had been let go. It occurred to me at the time that this could be the preliminary for a heart attack. But, being otherwise in good physical cardiovascular condition and active in strenuous activities, the pattern of ignoring other possible health conditions continued. The pattern of pacifying the subtle but ever-increasing symptoms were easily dismissed as "your just getting older" by the family physician, and an attempt to add a cholesterol inhibitor. This lasted for two months.

2005: Eighth Misdiagnosis—CHRONIC FATIGUE SYNDROME

Early in the fall of 2005, at the start of the new school year as network administrator for the Merrimack Valley School District, we were behind in getting lab and library computers setup. With more equipment ordered and no increase in staff, it was understood it would take some time into fall to be completely up and running. Everything was going wrong. Nothing worked right. Frustration and irritability rose in proportion. The problems requiring troubleshooting and analysis tripled. It seemed that the opposite of the Midas touch was newly acquired, as all efforts seemed mere fodder for Murphy's Law. And, it got worse. Even things that could not possibly go wrong started to. Every action seemed to require hours and hours of recovery time to fix the new problem just created from the old one. *And, I couldn't find things.* I would get to work without my cell phone, the next day my briefcase, the following day the pager, the day after that the phone *and* the briefcase.

There was not a day that went by without screaming at myself in the car on the way to work for mistakes and confusion about what, inexplicably, seemed to be impossible. The term for this is known as "Lyme rage," and it was used often by me as a form of self-punishment. Recurring pain in the knees was dismissed by the doctor as "Baker's Cysts." My feet felt as though they were plunged in ice-cold water year-round now. Further inability to concentrate or focus brought increases in Adderall. Persistent, severe anxiety and panic attacks were further subdued by increases in clonazepam. And just before Christmas vacation, while working on a computer lab in the middle-school, the level of frustration became so overpowering that I simply got up, left everything where it was and went home. I called the Superintendent's office and explained that I did not know when I would be back, and that this absence could be indefinite. They were very understanding. They knew that this was a highly visible and demanding position, that the pressures and responsibilities were enormous. They assured that the district would be fine, and to take as much time as I needed.

For the next four weeks, I sat by the wood stove and did not move or do anything except to eat and sleep, and keep the fire going. This feeling of being completely "stunned" was an ever-present and overwhelming manifestation of fear and panic. The feeling can be best described as a cornered animal, victimized by fear in a permanent desperate "fight-or-flight" condition of survival, and it had reduced me to complete incapacitation. The foreboding dark clouds that had threatened the horizons for years had finally come to roost, and I was lost in them, unable to find my way through or out of them. An all-pervasive fear was inescapable.

Paralyzed by utter despair and completely exhausted, finally, on

July 1, 2006, resignation as network administrator for the school district was inevitable, after ten years of steady employment. The day of reckoning had no goodbyes or farewells from the district for a job well done—nothing. No inquiries as to why. The letter of resignation expressed relief with having it over with, and the last few days worked out to leave one last time and never return. It was a big job with enormous responsibilities. Perhaps we all knew that the role could no longer be fulfilled, as incompetence triumphed. Upon taking the position in 1996, it was with the promise to never leave this job unless my position was terminated. It was a promise that could not be kept. Weary of the battle, there was nothing left to do but succumb to fatigue and complete despair. The specter of incapacity had overcome, and I had still had no idea why. As a result, Adderall was increased to compensate for the new and latest misdiagnosis—Chronic Fatigue Syndrome.

2007: Ninth Misdiagnosis—RHEUMATOID ARTHRITIS

At first, escaping to Belize became an obsession, followed by relocating to Florida. Though wearing wool socks year-round now, it felt like I was constantly standing in a pail of ice water. The "fight or flight" syndrome had become overwhelming and manifested itself permanently now as a new form of malignant PTSD. The feeling of suffocation, not getting enough air, breathing irregularly, all gave the sense of slow drowning. An overpowering feeling to start over, of changing identity or metamorphosing began around 2002. During these last years at the district before the premature "retirement," research of Belize as a new destination began, and developed into an escape plan. Four years later I got half the way there.

While researching the options, I followed up on a link to a job that oldest daughter Natalie had pointed out, with the recommendation accompanied by a comment something to the effect of "this might be what you're looking for." The description of the job ran basically as caretaker of a bamboo farm for a nudist family in central Florida. The terms were 20 hours per week in exchange for free rent living on the farm and being at least comfortable with the nudity part, if not willing to participate. After flying down Memorial Day Weekend in 2006 to try out for the position, we found it a match, and July 2nd was set as the first day—the first day after "retirement" from Merrimack Valley School District. The physical labor, the lack of complexity, being outdoors in the warm Florida sun, and having just one thing to do at a time—yes, multi-tasking skills were not required—all made the decision an overwhelming *yes*.

This attempt to establish a new identity, get into shape, and start over with a fresh new beginning proved effective at first but then quickly succumbed to utter disaster. There were many sublime moments of rapture in the garden on the bamboo farm, and new friends made were encouraging. After finding a psychiatrist in Leesburg FL, more benzo's, Cymbalta, and Adderall were prescribed. This new life had begun and went well for the next eight months, and new hope emerged in the Florida sunshine. That is, until one morning in April which I will never forget. With no strength left to lift up a mug of coffee that morning, because of extreme pain and weakness in the arms, my jaw would stop moving after chewing three bites. My short-lived tenure at the farm was suddenly doomed.

Just the day before, rolling 300-pound potted plants was no problem, but that morning widespread pain had gripped the arms, especially in the muscles, joints and tendons. The pain was excruciating; sometimes throbbing, sometimes radiating, sometimes shooting. It felt as if being electrocuted. It was a real struggle getting through that four-hour shift, and immediately a general practitioner was called for an appointment. The appointment set for two days later, it finally crossed my mind....

Could this be "Lyme?"

The doctor, genuinely puzzled and concerned over the symptoms, ordered a wide variety of lab tests to cover many possibilities. It became apparent that we must rule out Lyme, and so that test was also ordered. Days later, all tests were negative but for a slight indication of possible marker for rheumatoid arthritis. Though still seemingly perplexed, his recommendation was to see another specialist, this time a rheumatologist. And, so, the first Lyme test in 2007 came back as (or misdiagnosed as) *negative*, and the 9th misdiagnosis of rheumatoid arthritis began.

2008: Tenth Misdiagnosis—FIBROMYALGIA

By now, the whole body was engulfed in a kind of nerve pain that could be best described as electrical interference. Not only did everyday vision resemble a fluorescent light flickering as a symptom of pending failure, the arms felt like they were being electrocuted; like the fingers were stuck in electrical wall outlets. The rheumatologist assured that there was "nothing that can be done" for the condition except treating symptoms. It was permanent and incurable, but not progressive, and that with treatment you can still maintain some quality of life. The chronic disease missed all these years he diagnosed as "*fibromyalgia*." Little did I know at the time, this diagnosis is a dumping ground for people in my condition, who are considered hopeless, a hypochondriac, a malingerer with a psychosomatic illness of unknown origin.

Sure enough, here come new meds—Lyrica for the pain, Amytriptiline for dysautonomia. Amitriptyline is a tricyclic antidepressant that is widely used to treat chronic neuropathic pain due to nerve damage, fibromyalgia and dysautonomia. Dysautonomia, or autonomic dysfunction, is a condition in which the autonomic nervous system does not work properly. This may affect the functioning of the heart, bladder, intestines, sweat glands, pupils, and blood vessels. Cymbalta for severe pain resulting from depression. Prozac was added for bi-polar depression, Clonazepam for the crippling anxiety, and Adderall for the profound chronic fatigue.

Back in 30 days.

The rheumatologist ordered more tests. Suspicions being raised again, at this point another Lyme test was demanded. This had to be fought for, as the rheumatologist strongly discouraged getting the test. "*If you do have it, the cost can be in the thousands of dollars*," he emphasized. As if that made a *difference*? I was incredulous. Why would anyone not want to know for sure? Perplexed, I nonetheless demanded the test against his admonishments to forego it. We needed to know for sure that it was not Lyme. Results of Lyme Test #2 were, once again, *negative*.

Incompetence finally triumphed. The end of 2008 ended in severe widespread pain and complete incapacitation. Now disabled and nearly completely paralyzed, any movement was virtually impossible. Having drawn upon all available resources, all were sacrificed for the "good cause." During the real estate bust of 2008, the income properties would not sell and were threatened with foreclosure. Meanwhile, experienced at random times was a peculiar form of *involuntarily shutdown*. Seemingly at the most inopportune times, the body would randomly just stop working, like a computer involuntarily powering down from an exhausted battery. Wherever I was at the time, I would have to pull off the road while driving, or climb into the backseat of the car to crash while out doing errands, for anywhere from 10 minutes to half an hour. Brains zaps, jolts, jerks, tics, spasms, twitches—there seemed to be no end to the random stream of symptoms, and no established pattern whatsoever. Most all the time, the feeling of being electrocuted was constant. The pain—*excruciating*. And still simmering in the back of the mind, a whispering voice questioned the possibility:

Could this be Lyme?

Socially more and more withdrawn, relationships disappeared, friends faded away, and isolation became the norm. The ability to interact with other people and communicate effectively was all but gone except at a very basic level. Solitary confinement realized, which had been progressively getting worse for many years, it became clear that it would not be long before total incoherence was inevitable, and the ability to care for myself impossible.

There were more trips to the emergency room with episodes of extreme panic attacks, severe pain and psychosis. I moved back to New Hampshire in 2009 in an attempt to save the house we had built on the Blackwater River from foreclosure. Already lost were the other real estate investments, and bankruptcy was looking like the only option. Resources dwindled, food stamps denied, health care denied, life became a constant state of denial and fear. Heat from the wood stove that winter was mostly supplied by old furniture collected that day from the landfill station, with legs and arms sawed off those old chairs committed to the flames. Definitely not the same person anymore, more an empty shell that had ceased to exit, it occurred to me—*am I even human anymore*?

2009: Final Diagnosis—NEURO-BORRELIOSIS

Upon returning to Florida in late 2009, after foreclosure and bankruptcy, it was as if by a vanquished knight in tarnished armor, dull blade, dented, broken shield, and fatigued by battle from slaying many dragons of my own creation. Attempts to become re-established were short-lived, and some time was spent jumping between Beverly Hills, Spring Hill and Floral City, all in the general Citrus County area of the central mid-west coast of Florida, just north of Tampa. An attempt to adapt new skills as an antique furniture re-finisher were compromised, as only an hour or two per day of useful productive time did not go far enough. With small seizures, Parkinson-like tremors, speech impediments, and Tourette-like outbursts, it was becoming clear that the time was coming soon where continuing would be impossible.

An upcoming appointment with a Social Security Disability attorney in Tampa was the last-ditch effort. There was neither the strength nor the will anymore to continue, and the first thing said to the attorney upon the first visit was,

"This is the end of the road."

At that time, there seemed only four choices: nursing home, prison, hospice, or death. The attorney was reassuring and made me promise to keep seeing the doctor, stay away from drugs (the "bad" ones), and stay alive. By Christmas, it was evident that the time had come to admit I was completely disabled. Great humility learned that night, it was clear that incompetence had claimed victory. Doing anything wasn't even in the vocabulary anymore, as waves of anxiety and dementia continued to spiral out of control. A rescue mission was formed by my mother, for me, who at 49 years of age was unable to function.

How much worse could this possibly get?

My mother was one of several "angels" that appeared during this time of need. She gave me life twice: once when I was born, and again at forty-nine years old when she demanded "*You're getting another Lyme test—only this time with IGeneX—and you are not going to argue with me about this*!" Despite earlier attempts to deflect her advice, I had no strength or will to prevail, and plans commenced for a flight from Tampa to Manchester, NH where she had arranged an appointment with someone experienced in treating patients with Lyme.

Christmas came and went, and the appointment loomed ominous. This time, Angel #2 appeared in my life—a Lyme literate nurse practitioner, or LLMD (Lyme-literate doctor), who gave it to me straight. Based on the evidence of the symptoms alone, she believed according to her clinical diagnosis there existed a 90%+ chance of having the disease, but that the lab tests through IGeneX, who claim a 95% accuracy rate (high above the norm of other labs like LabCorp and Quest) would verify this. I told the doctor that if this is indeed the case I would build a shrine to my mother for leading me here. The doctor replied that I should start saving my money for it now, given the high probability. Blood was drawn at the office, and I was sent home to wait the 7 to 10-day lab response.

The hour was getting late, indeed.

Never will be forgotten the day and moment that the phone call with the truth arrived.

Diagnosis confirmed: ***late-stage, advanced Neuroborreliosis****.*
Advanced, late-stage Lyme disease.

"You have evidence of 'old' Lyme," the doctor explained on the phone. The next appointment was made to obtain several antibiotic prescriptions; Biaxin (clarythromycin) and Plaquenil (hydroxychloroquine). The doctor continued to be frank about the rough road ahead. She explained that treatment would cause a "herx" reaction, a result of inflammation from severe die-off of the spirochete that would be experienced as worse than the disease itself. And, that this was going to take a *long time*. How long? Months. Maybe years. The doctor was good about setting the terms and expectations for recovery, and reassured that recovery was probable if the program was strictly adhered to. With the highly acclaimed and controversial Lyme documentary "*Under Our Skin*" as part of the first week of treatment, we obtained a copy of the DVD and began to learn the hard truth about Lyme, and the many myths that perpetuate the frequent misunderstandings about this disease.

It was obvious that the days ahead were going to be the most difficult of all to date. And there were no guarantees. But one thing was certain: *there was nothing to lose*. Everything once earned, saved, deserved, owned, acquired, achieved, obtained, maintained or desired were gone. Even the faculties of reason and will were gone. There was only one possible direction left to be considered; forward.

As promised, the shrine to my mother began. A fountain, garden angels, solar lights were assembled in the backyard in the corner by the house. To this day I have a shrine also in my own home dedicated to her.

PART 2:

Enduring the Path to Well-Being

Desperation.

Anger.

Fear.

Dread.

Frustration.

The symptoms were *excruciating*; the ordeal seemed hopeless. Having finally tested positive after so many years and two false negative tests, treatment began immediately. The powerful antibiotic Biaxin (clarithromycin) at 500mg and the anti-parasitic Plaquenil (hydroxychloroquine) at 200mg was administered twice daily for the next thirty-six months. The side effects began a nightmare of relentless pain and agony, and with it a desperate yearning for relief. There was no detectable progress noted during the first twenty-four months, just an ebb and flow of worsening and improving conditions, some days seeing some slight improvement and relief, others seeing relapse into the depths of hell. The pharmaceuticals already prescribed for symptoms became "temporary helpers" along the way; the only true friends left.

Words cannot truly describe the experience of surviving treatment. Being tortured 24/7 by electrocution and pain comes to mind, as does clinging to a buoy in the middle of a turbulent ocean during a typhoon. That buoy is called "hope," and the dogged determination to cling to it is called "will." And, both were tested beyond the capacity for it. When one has been relieved of all once held dear, there remains a faith that one day again the sun will shine, all that is good will return, and with it the person that originally embarked on that journey. All true, but for the latter. The original person did not return, but one transformed by the experience.

Regardless of having the appearance of being otherwise healthy and normal, for anyone in the late stages of advanced Lyme disease, doing anything can often be an unrealistic challenge. Similar to a stroke victim, performing simple tasks we take for granted—like eating, dressing,

showering, even just breathing—can become huge challenges, if not impossible. Speech, communication, and reasoning can become severely impaired.

The role of a LLMD (Lyme-Literate-Medical-Doctor) is a primary requirement in the recovery of the patient. In addition, the probability of recovery assumes these additional three roles, as critical to increasing the chances of "saving" someone with Lyme:

(1) a LLMD;

(2) an Advocate;

(3) a Caretaker;

(4) a Benefactor.

1) Finding a Lyme-literate Medical Doctor (LLMD)

The importance of finding the services of a Lyme-literate doctor or LLMD is essential. An important additional point and distinction must be made here to distinguish between two philosophies of treatment, when it comes to which LLMD to accept as your primary care giver. The further qualification for finding the right LLMD is to ensure you select one who embraces the treatment philosophy of ILADS, as opposed to IDSA, guidelines for treatment. You will want to select a LLMD who subscribes to the ILADS guidelines for treatment. ILADS stands for *International Lyme and Associated Diseases Society*. This group of Lyme-literate doctors (the ILADS group) understand the positive implications of long-term antibiotic treatment as highly probable for recovery and often necessary for complete remission of the patient.

Contrarily, the IDSA (Infections Disease Society of America) observes strict guidelines for antibiotic treatment that *do not exceed* 30-days in duration. An infectious disease doctor or specialist who subscribes to the principles of treatment under the IDSA guidelines is unlikely to observe the evidence of long-term antibiotic treatment. Infectious disease doctors of the IDSA group strictly adhere to the guidelines of limiting patients to a *maximum* 30-day limit of antibiotics, which has proven ineffective in curing late-stage advanced Lyme disease patients. You will want to find a LLMD who is willing to get you to the finish line, no matter how long it takes (ILADS, *not* ISDA.) This increases the probability of a full recovery, without relapse.

LLMD's are rare and can be hard to find. Often a Lyme support group in your area will have contact information for how to find one or more in your area. Other online groups such as ilads.org, lymediseaseassociation.org and others are good sources for referrals for finding a LLMD who is ILADS compliant. Simple online internet searches will reveal these links and others and guide you to someone in your area. Keep in mind that these doctors are often highly sought after and have long waiting times for new patients. You may also have to drive great distances to find one available that will meet your objectives, qualifications and time-frame.

It is often the case that LLMDs will only accept cash as payment, as most insurance carriers refuse to recognize Lyme as a legitimate disease eligible for coverage. These are some of the hard truths about getting well again, but they must be overcome at all costs. This is where the help of an Advocate and/or Benefactor can make a huge difference.

2) Finding an Advocate

An Advocate is someone close to the patient who oversees that general care is properly conducted and concluded. With oversight and benevolence, this individual "keeps the ball rolling" in the right direction. The Advocate's role is to ensure that there is a LLMD in place for treatment, that a Caretaker is appointed to care for the patient during treatment if necessary, and that a Benefactor is available to assist with the financial care of the patient if required. It is sometimes the role of the Advocate to assist in one or all three of these areas, and in some cases takes responsibility for all three roles. A spouse, parent, close friend, son, or daughter may inevitably fulfill one or all these roles.

3) Finding a Caretaker

The Caretaker has one priority—to help the patient get well again on a date-to-day basis. Often these roles are played by a single person; a parent, sibling or friend–who bares the brunt of the care-taking while the patient begins the long journey home to well-being. Tasks of the Caretaker include making sure that the prescribed medications are taken consistently, meals are prepared, and doctor visits made. This might also include shopping, socializing and entertainment needs are met, in order to improve the quality of treatment as much as possible.

4) Finding a Benefactor

If the patient is unable to work or has not prevailed with Medicare or Social Security Disability, there is increased chance of full recovery with a Benefactor. As most insurance carriers refuse to acknowledge the existence of or recognize Lyme disease as a legitimate illness, denial of care multiplies the cost of getting well. As a result, LLMDs do not accept most insurance plans, as their prescribed care will not be covered by insurance. For many, if not most, this seems like an insurmountable obstacle to getting the care required. Most people are strapped for the cash necessary to proceed with treatment and are faced with sacrificing property and financial assets prematurely. It is all the more difficult for the young or financially destitute.

There are no easy answers to these difficulties. But one thing is certain–*the required financial burdens of treatment must be met in order to recover.* One cannot get there by deciding to continue to pay off credit card or even mortgage obligations in lieu of getting treatment. Frequently, foreclosure and bankruptcy are the method by which the once fortunate become well again, as was my case. Faced with the choice between saving one's house from foreclosure or becoming well again is never an easy one, but it is often the necessary path for those with no other choice. When it comes to financing the cost of treatment, there is a deep, dark and sinister "Darwinian" struggle that unfolds, characteristic of the struggle against the disease itself. Only the strong and the financially capable survive, or the lucky. Short of a miracle itself, the odds are often stacked against the victim, and as unfair as this seems, it is the reality behind this devastating ordeal. With the onset of gradually decreasing capabilities, an Advocate, Caretaker, or Benefactor can increase the probability of making it to the finish line versus proceeding on one's own.

Lyme is a humbling experience. There is no shame or guilt in being sick, but it is often experienced by the afflicted. Once proud bread-winners, talented artists, educated businessmen, devoted mom's, or exemplary students—when these faculties are robbed of us, we feel cheated, forlorn and forsaken by life. No longer capable of fending for ourselves, humility has its day, and we succumb of necessity to assistance and support from others. Family and friends are often the only choice. Organizations and public programs like Food Stamps, Welfare and Disability can help. Private organizations that offer assistance might include churches or social organizations for the homeless and veterans. Though perhaps not a desired choice, such programs are available. Accept your blessings humbly, knowing that in the end you will pay it forward. These programs exist to make it possible. Being a receiver of benefits is not "taking." It is our time to accept the gifts and blessing that exist for that reason. It is our time to receive, knowing that this is the key not just to survival, but necessary to once again give back.

PART 3

Testimony from the Journey: Through the Labyrinth of Despair

2010: Surviving Treatment—"Am I Getting Better or Worse?"

The first night on Biaxin and Plaquenil seemed like it would be my last. The pain emanating from the area of the heart and the struggle to keep breathing was such that sleeping on the left side was completely avoided for the first several nights, for fear the extra strain would make the heart explode. The level of heart, brain, and central nervous system involvement was *pervasive*. Pain in the joints, muscles, tendons, fingers, knuckles, wrists, and elbows became excruciating, sometimes beyond the point of intolerable. Followed by worsening conditions of PTSD, Parkinson's, Alzheimer's, multiple sclerosis, dementia, depersonalization, dysautonomia. The list grew, and it was often questioned whether the condition was getting better or worse.

Was the tide coming in or going out?
Or, both at the same time?
It was impossible to tell in the short run.

Everyone who has Lyme manifests its own laundry list of rotating symptoms. Depending on when and where the infection occurred, and under what circumstances it spread, there exists a multitude of symptoms that manifest in different ways. Certainly the muscles, joints and tendons can be severely affected, as with the nerve endings in the spine, central nervous system and brain. Some studies reveal over 300 different symptoms that can be attributed to the disease, many of which overlap, disappear, then reappear later down the road.

There is an endless choice of supplements that are out there for every ache and ailment under the sun, and anyone with an unlimited financial resources can amuse and distract themselves indefinitely, but the real dogs gnawing on the root of the problem are always the *antibiotics*. Yes, diet, vitamins and moderate exercise are all important towards a balanced approach to help boost the immune system, but without the *consistent duration of antibiotics (abx)* the chances of overcoming the disease is severely reduced. The effects of recovery, even with the help of numerous supplements, are nonetheless brutal and excruciating. Dementia sets in. There is no reason. There is no will. There is no *identity*. And the *will to live* is severely diminished.

The ordeal has a dehumanizing effect. The faculties that make us human disappear. I recall screaming at my doctor,

"I don't even know if I am human anymore!"

I described my experience to the doctor. Being hit by severe waves of absolute terror and dementia every twenty minutes, it was like being lost and submerged in the ocean during a violent storm with no life preserver; just a rock to cling to until the next wave hit, knocking me back into the dark cold waters threatening imminent death.

You think a lot about Death. It's hard not to dwelling in the face of it, barely able to hold it off. You come to question whether or not it's the better answer—or the *only* answer. It would be so much easier… Then, I would crawl back up on that rock, barely hanging on, and brace for the next inevitable wave.

In telling the doctor about the *fear*—a deep, dark, penetrating fear of ominous foreboding and dread—Amitriptyline was gradually increased tenfold. And more. Next, a Tourette-like symptom began to impair my speech.

The horror of surviving the ordeal of recovery will test the endurance of even the strongest person. Not only will you have to give up trying to do most things you used to enjoy, but learn to accept, learn to be comfortable with, and perhaps even embrace *doing nothing*. The number of long hours endured, minute by minute, second by second, laying still with eyes closed, unable to move—this is more than most people can bear. Going the route of the Buddhist monk, accepting fate, and adapting to a life of meditation offered the only way to endure this long dark "night of the soul."

Being perfectly comfortable in a meditative state for hours doing absolutely nothing is the greatest gift of Lyme. It is the one and only peaceful place that can be claimed to exist during the entire ordeal. The rest of the struggle was otherwise often accompanied by thoughts of hopelessness, utter despair, or even suicide. Eventually there came a time when a very peculiar *sensation of a separation of mind and body* became increasingly apparent. The loss of *temporal-spatial* sensation was dramatic. The sense of continuity of time itself no longer existed. Dates, times, and places ceased to exist in a real sense. Often it was not known what day of the week it was, or even what month. It seemed that time began anew each day, the slate was wiped clean. I was literally born again each day upon waking up.

The three-dimensional world all but disappeared. Being in public became an ordeal, bumbling and fumbling along, walking in front of people, getting in the way, bumping into things unseen. Constantly being in the way was humiliating to say the least. Trips to the grocery store were living nightmares to get through and were not a good reason to get out. The isolation, the withdrawal from living itself, is a form of solitary confinement that is neither self-imposed or projected by others. The overwhelming feeling was not so much "get me out of here" as "*you do not belong here.*" It is part of a horrendous secondary existence, the *Lymelands* as described in Pamela Weintraub's recent book "*Cure Unknown.*" Lyme rage, hopelessness and despair continue in a downward spiral, and there is no controlling it. It's not a matter of looking at the problem correctly, seeing it in the right light, and that the cup is half full as the psychiatrists and psychologists had told me for years. The cup was not full or empty, there was no cup. Period.

With absolutely nothing that can be done, the only thing left is to let the abx do its work and wait, be patient, and ride it out. Let the glacier move at its own pace; the terrapin make its way across the desert; the snail along the sidewalk. It is not a sprint to the finish line, it is a long-distance run that requires pacing one's self accordingly. There are no shortcuts, no silver bullets, no magical incantations or divine interventions. Just slow, steady progress, one step in front of the other, every second an eternity in itself, plodding, wading, resting, clawing, crawling and scraping one's way through the abysmal Swamp of Despair.

Am I getting better or worse?

As if having the disease is not enough, the Herxheimer effect—caused by the abx treatment—of toxins inflaming and invading the body's tissues is doubly cruel. The die-off of the Borrelia Burgdorferi spirochete exacerbates the symptoms, making the ordeal intolerable. Time crawls on like a slug for days, weeks, months, with seemingly no progress, no recognizable pattern, just random attacks that come and go. Every day there was the threatening notion that the protocol must not be working, as there is no real apparent progress from one day to the next. A constant impulse to change the protocol, change doctors or just give up becomes a daily struggle. It takes *duration of time* to know whether the tide is still coming in or going out.

When you can no longer trust your judgment about such things, *everything* you think is suspect. What is "real" and what is just another Lyme-induced hallucination? Distortion of perception is a frequent peril of Lymers. Trust—in anything—disappears under the horizon of the past. Life itself is fading away, replaced by a state of Purgatory that even Dante would struggle to articulate.

2011: Enduring the Journey Through the "Swamp"—A Life or Death Struggle

The journey back to Normal will test your will and endurance long after both are gone. But, now there is no choice. You're in for the long haul.... it's too late now to turn back. Turning back is not an option, as that option is the final one: death. Or *worse*. One learns that there are things about life that are worse than death. Death is so easy compared to living in a perpetual hell. Now squarely in the middle of the Swamp, there is no turning back, there is no rest, only moving inch by inch with the speed of a glacier through the muck that has you mired waist deep. To stop is to sink, to go back is to die, but what could be worse than death?

To have endured Lyme is to know that there are things worse than death.

To live and endure such misery is akin to torture, 24/7. No wonder so many on this journey give up. The rates of suicide reveal it as the number one cause of death amongst the afflicted. This is not difficult to understand for an advanced late-stage Lymer. It is a rare occurrence that one makes it all the way through the Swamp, to crawl out on the banks on the other side and experience the sun once again—to stand, to walk, to speak from one's mind that has been miraculously restored from the dungeon of silence. It is in a real sense Darwinian–*only the strong survive*. To reach the Promised Land of Normal again is all that Lymers dream of; the great day of resolve, of resurrection, of a new life again in the face of bleak and weary and seemingly endless struggle. It is the dream of *living again* that is the one driving force that pushes back against the cruelty and despair that threatens every day, every hour, every minute, every second. For students of psychology who confront the phrase "there is no such thing as normal" there is definitely such a thing to the Lymer. To be Normal again is the Holy Grail, the end of the long, tortuous quest, the one goal that keeps the dream alive is the promise to actually live again. Is it Atonement? Are Lymers on the path to some kind of spiritual Redemption?

To say that the struggle is Darwinian in nature, that only the strong prevail, that it is survival of the fittest–this is difficult to say but even more difficult to question or argue with. It can be compared to the one single spermatozoa that makes the journey all the way up the uterine canal to unite with the egg; or the salmon that overcomes great adversity to find its way home from ocean vastness up the small stream of its origin, the primordial home of its ancestors. There are many suitable analogies to describe the journey to Normal, to be home again, where Paradise awaits and once more rewards the courageous, the bold, the defiant, the strong–and the lucky.

There seems to be an undeniable element of luck. And sacrifice. Being in the right place at the right time, finding an Advocate, finding the right LLMD, a Caretaker, having the necessary finances; it seems that these all must occur in the right sequence, in the right order, at the right time, for everything to be *just right* for the Lymer to find their way out of the Swamp, back to the Promised Land, and succeed. Is it a matter of perseverance and determination, plain dumb luck, or divine intervention? Or is it all of the above?

A peculiar idiosyncrasy of this disease compares to the shameful stigma and shunning of the "leper" of ancient times. This shunning by our modern society, the shameful denial, the deliberate ignorance committed by the medical community—to turn away from the cries of the afflicted, to deny insurance, to ignore the causes—this mis-treatment of the afflicted echoes the calls of the "unclean" shouted by the Lepers of old to warn others.

Another particular idiosyncrasy in the mis-treatment of this disease is considering it a "moral" crime. People "convicted" of Lyme are treated like criminals, like they are somehow responsible for their own crime of affliction and therefore have incurred the punishment they deserve. The stigma attached to Lyme is further exacerbated by the media; the lack of exposure and coverage in the news, the isolation and obscuration of the very *existence* of these phenomena. It begs the question, "what *is it* about Lyme?" It begs of conspiracy, deliberate cover-up, of saving face, and, most obviously now, denial, denial, denial....

The prevailing attitude toward Lyme is one that people don't want to hear about it. They simply refuse to recognize, acknowledge or accept it as a possibility for themselves or others. The stigmas of mental illness, accusations of hypochondria, malingerers, that it is all about ones "attitude" or "all just in your head" are frequently echoed from the doctor's office, the media, the CDC, IDSA, and the medical community in general. To deflect blame, the deniers accuse the legions of the afflicted, that they deserve their punishment, and somehow deserve to be hidden in shame behind the prison walls of their own demise, away from view, swept under the rug. Even our closest family members, loved ones and dearest friends often deny the existence of any real problem in favor of "faking" the dilemma, for attention, out of laziness, or just plain giving up on themselves.

Because it is hidden behind this general haze of denial it has been permitted to creep across the threshold of nearly every household, while the public remains mesmerized and distracted by anything and everything under the sun but the truth about Lyme. Thereby rendered unable to react to this imminent danger, we carefully avoid confronting this invisible intruder as the public continues to pretend that it doesn't exist. This kind of self-incrimination is not just about Lyme, but at the heart of all human misery and suffering.

Wading through the muck of the Primordial Swamp that the Lymer must endure, in addition to an already overwhelming disease that cripples the ability to withstand, it is against staggering odds that anyone who enters this Swamp ever emerges victorious on the other side. This is not meant to discourage those who enter, but a warning to the unaware or unprepared. Beware those with good intentions who encourage Lyme patients to "take a break" from treatment, their doctor in particular. This is a frequent cause of relapse and failure of treatment, and those who do this usually find themselves back at the beginning of the Swamp. Also, beware the well-meaning advice of those who purport so-called "natural" cures. Though these claims are made with good heart and intention, there exists a real possibility that the Borrelia spirochete has been scientifically tampered with. Given this possibility as the first genetically modified organism (GMO), there is a high probability that:

"It may take science to undo what science has created."

So, when you begin treatment, don't stop. This simply cannot be overemphasized. And once you start, don't look back, and don't stop. On through the Swamp, keep moving forward, and don't look back!

2012: Trapped in a "Glass Terrarium"

Victims of advanced late-stage Lyme may find themselves isolated socially, or confined to bed, even virtually paralyzed, almost completely unable to move. It is small wonder that these are often misdiagnosed with multiple sclerosis, Parkinson's, ALS, Lupus, or the myriad of other neuro-skeletal or neuro-muscular conditions. Feeling trapped within a crippled body is often similar to victims of stroke or even heart disease, where confinement and isolation render the patient helpless in taking care of themselves.

This slow demise into solitary confinement can be described as being trapped behind a glass wall, stuck in a dreary terrarium, the glass smudged and stained, making it difficult to see out into the everyday world of ordinary life. Completely cut off from society and humanity in general, unable to interact or even communicate with one's own kind, the hard truth is not often discussed. Socially untidy, it does not seem appropriate and not something one generally wishes to be exposed to.

Understandably, the generally healthy would prefer to remain in this oblivious state of denial about the truth behind Lyme. That is, until it invades your own body, or that of a loved one. Hence the saying about Lyme:

"You don't get it 'til you've got it."

This is, after all, a natural reaction to affliction from the non-afflicted. It is a form of natural instinct to thrive when you are healthy. In most all other cases of disease the sick and infirmed are ignored and hidden from view of the public. Unaware of the known four possible means of transmission, the public goes about their business as if all is well, nothing is wrong, blind to the danger at the doorstep.

And yet, it is a natural tendency for otherwise healthy human beings to go about their daily business in the safety and comfort of denial, suppressing potential threats to their own well-being. A normal defense mechanism that presents all living organisms with the opportunity to flourish, these forms of denial prevent the complete breakdown of societal forms of organization and interaction. On the other hand, denial can exude blindness that ignores the gradual signs and symptoms that, if continued, could dangerously overwhelm and devastate health and destroy well-being.

In the natural cycles of birth, growth and death, the spontaneous generation, decline, recovery, and the eventual decay of all organisms is an immutable law of nature, one that can only be prolonged or delayed. The inevitable consequences of suffering are practically non-existent to the daily consciousness of the living while we thrive, and only recognized when in a state of decline. It is no small wonder that early symptoms of Lyme are ignored, and routinely denied or suppressed. But, at what point does one recognize the inherent danger? The boiling-frog example best describes this human proclivity. The slow advancement of increasing water temperature goes unnoticed by the frog who entered the pot when the water was cool, until it is too late and the frog boils. In contrast, a frog that suddenly finds itself in hot water will be aware of the danger and leap from the pot to safety. There are no clear-cut solutions to this, as seen in the chronology of the slow, stealthy manifestation of the disease that is realized too late. There is no steaming hot, obvious symptom that signals a need to act. Often no bulls-eye rash manifests at the original onset of Lyme disease, contrary to popular belief fueled by decades of mis-information by the medical community. By the time symptoms of late-stage advanced Lyme are present, the frog has already been boiled alive. Certainly, catching it early starts with awareness, followed by recognition, acknowledgment, acceptance, and finally followed by action-based solutions.

2012: The Lyme Cure—Antibiotic Treatment vs. Natural Remedies

Increasingly, people are turning to natural remedies in seeking treatment for Lyme disease. A holistic approach toward healing is gaining ground *in the face of* established medical science, especially for those who have not obtained relief from a standard 30-day course of antibiotics. There is growing evidence that a holistic approach can help provide relief from the relentless ebb and flow of symptoms associated with the disease and can be an important part of the overall treatment of inflammation resulting from antibiotic treatment. As many Lyme victims claim failure from antibiotic treatment, usually resulting from premature discontinuation, more often they seek alternative medicine to best support their decision to abandon antibiotic treatment in favor of learning to live with the disease.

The cure for Lyme is often a complex one, requiring so-called "supplements" which include everything from vitamins, diet and natural remedies, to pharmaceuticals necessary to control and relieve the many symptoms of depression, anxiety, fatigue and pain.

- Natural supplements also combine to boost the immune system.
- Consumption of sugar, wheat and dairy are discouraged by some Lyme-literate medical doctors, suggesting that not only does the spirochete feed on these, but these foods tend to exacerbate inflammation during the recovery process, particularly in the gut.
- Because antibiotics kill bacteria indiscriminately, the good with the bad, pro-biotics are frequently recommended to offset the destruction of "good" bacteria necessary for proper digestion.
- Given that yogurt contains the bacteria we need to regulate digestion but is a dairy product, fermented foods like sauerkraut contain many times more the number of microbes needed and are a good source of pro-biotic.

There are several primary reasons why patients give up on antibiotic treatment and, as a result, abandon their best chance for a true cure. Though treatment can be undeniably excruciating, the victim often is not in the best position to determine what needs to be done. By the time the disease has compromised the brain, central nervous system, and the heart and muscle tissues, there is a desperation for relief that is overpowering, and this tends to cloud judgment. In this way, the desperation for relief can lead to self-defeating behavior.

Here is why:

1) The number one reason that patients give up antibiotic treatment in favor of natural remedies is that they cannot endure the excruciating symptoms of inflammation that results from the die-off of the Borrelia spirochete called a "Herx" reaction. The Jarisch–Herxheimer reaction is due to endotoxins released by the death of harmful microorganisms like Borrelia within the body during antibiotic treatment. First discovered by dermatologists Adolf Jarisch and Karl Herxheimer, while treating Syphilis, (another closely related spirochete and probable progenitor of the modern Lyme spirochete Borrelia) it resembles bacterial sepsis and can occur after initiation of antibacterials. After several weeks of treatment, when the normal expectation of feeling better does not materialize, the natural response by the patient is that the treatment must not be working.

This is far from the truth.

Extremely counter-intuitive to the typical experience of antibiotics, where after a few days the symptoms begin to subside, the continued presence of a high misery index actually means the antibiotic treatment is *still doing its job—continued suffering is a sign there are still microorganisms present in the body*. In fact, the negative reaction to antibiotic treatment is how a good LLMD will clinically measure progress of treatment.

However, as the weeks or months drag on with no relief, the patient wrestles with the specter of doubt about whether the treatment is working. Added pressure in the absence of real change leads the patient and/or the doctor to give up treatment prematurely, and for a while the patient feels better. But inevitably, the symptoms return, and the process starts over. The vicious cycle is repeated, and actually lengthens the time required to become free of the disease. An example cited is that of baking a potato. Is it done yet? Is the temperature high enough? Has it been in long enough? If the antibiotic level is not strong enough, and treatment not long enough, the potato (the patient) is not "done" yet. You want to be "fully baked," and then some, to be sure.

2) The second most frequent reason for abandoning antibiotics in favor of natural remedies is *an insufficient duration of treatment.* While 30-days of antibiotic treatment is usually the standard of treatment for Lyme cases that are caught immediately after infection, such as those cases reported with a bulls-eye tick bite, the maximum of 30-days is often woefully inadequate for those diagnosed with late-stage disseminated Lyme disease. Once Lyme has been in the body for an extended period of time, the spirochetes have infested farther and deeper into the tissues, organs, nervous system and brain. For the chronically ill, treatment can more often take many months to several years before the patient sees real progress. This is where the importance of holistic medicine plays an important role, in boosting the immune system and abating the severity of symptoms during treatment. However, the use of holistic medicine *alone* in combating Lyme disease, in the absence of treatment with antibiotics, is rarely sufficient for ridding the body of the spirochete.

Beware the well-meaning claims of a natural or holistic cure without antibiotics.

It is one thing to seek and hope for a miracle, quite another to ignore the science behind such a miracle. Take the supplements, the vitamins, the herbal remedies, and any or all of the other purported fixes, but *keep science gnawing on the root of the problem*, which at least for now, is long-term antibiotic treatment—for as long as it takes.

There is a prevailing attitude amongst some holistic doctors that there is a "natural cure" for all maladies and diseases. These are well-meaning, but possibly misguided, healers who can derail your path to success. They may be correct in the sense that natural healing through herbs and diet can eradicate natural diseases, but the reasoning may be seriously deficient if the disease is not caused by nature, but *caused by science*. On the side of caution due to the possibility that Borrelia has been inadvertently or otherwise "tweaked" genetically to avoid human immune response, again:

It may require science to cure what science has created.

This supports the pattern that is observed over and over in the success of long-term treatment with antibiotics, compared with the opposite of near certain relapse when the patient abandons antibiotic therapy in favor of the natural path. **Once on the antibiotic protocol, *stay the course.*** We are at all times dealing here with probabilities, and one can only increase or decrease the probability of success. Continue to take whatever supplements necessary, natural or pharmaceutical, but *do not abandon the course of antibiotics*. Deviations from this path, in most observable and clinical cases, reveals the probability of relapse, and recovering from relapse is made all the more difficult.

3) The third and most prevalent reason against long-term antibiotic treatment is doctors themselves, who are instructed it is in their own best interest to discourage the "overuse" of antibiotics. Often touting that such abuse leads to mutations of pathogens that resist treatment, this has led doctors to develop an overwhelming bias against long-term antibiotics, even when warranted by what would otherwise present as obvious persistent infection.

2013: The Four-fold Path to Remission—How A Cure Is Possible

The diagram on the next page depicts the four (4) major steps that make it possible to survive Lyme, and increase the probability of a full remission. Essentially, any deviation from this map to recovery leads to the "still-critically-ill" category of so many Lyme casualties. The path to becoming well again is both a labyrinth and a gauntlet and going astray severely decreases the possibility of discovery and treatment. Because of this, the impact on the severely afflicted in deviating from this path can lead to devastating long-term consequences.

This suggests that the reality of Lyme in the present day is far from turning the tide to victory. Far too many are still overlooked, ignored, or denied and, as a result, left behind in the hands of the so-called "specialists." Given the widespread nature of Lyme disease and it's many manifestations, and so often misdiagnosed as one of the many chronic illnesses that plague our society today, when someone decides to get tested for Lyme, consider these four important principles:

(1) The first and most important step is *finding a Lyme-literate doctor*, often referred to as a LLMD. Finding a good LLMD as the first step on the Four-fold Path is the biggest obstacle to overcome on your way to becoming well again. A good LLMD will diagnose your condition clinically, but will also have your blood tested at the IGeneX Lab in Palo Alto, California. Be sure your LLMD is associated with ILADS. Beware doctors associated with the IDSA who strictly adhere to a maximum limit of not more than thirty (30) days of antibiotics treatment. IDSA doctors typically deny patients long-term antibiotic treatment.

HOW TO SURVIVE LYME DISEASE

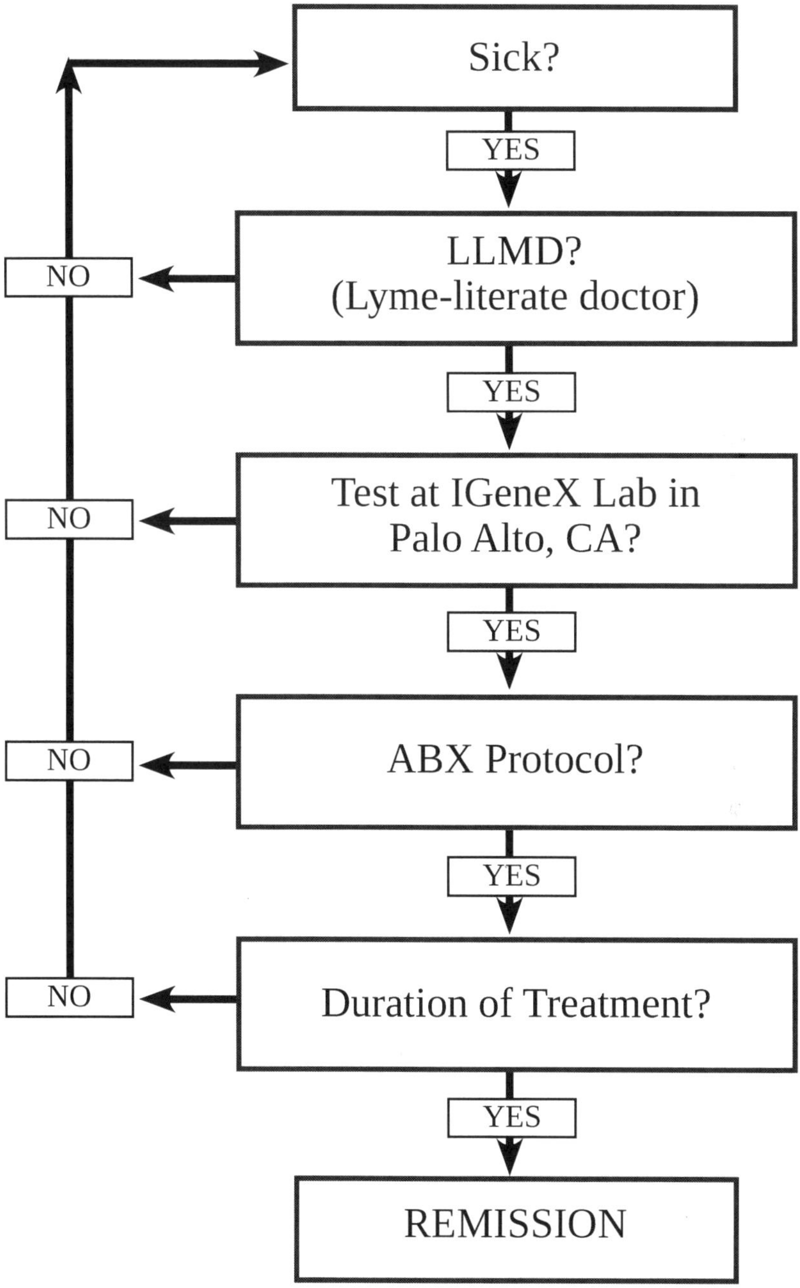

2) Getting tested at the *__IGeneX Lab__* in Palo Alto, CA. The IGeneX Lab has a higher accuracy rate than any other available labs such as Quest or Labcorp, when detecting Lyme disease that has been in the body for a long time. Common labs have notoriously poor track records of false negatives, by some estimates more than three out of five or more. This has caused great harm to many people, and remains one of the biggest issues in successfully combating Lyme disease. If a person is not diagnosed, they cannot be treated. Additional screenings for co-infections such as bartonella, babesia, mycoplasma, ehrlichia, etc. can also be ordered through IGeneX. And yes, the tests at IGeneX are expensive. But, would you rather pay $50 for a test that comes back as a false negative and lose your ability to work, your house, car and way of life, or pay $500 for a test that is accurate and puts you on the road to recovery? Which is *actually* more expensive? **This is not the time to look for ways to save money on becoming healthy again.** It may be the most important investment you ever make! Trying to save money at this point would be akin to stiffing the waiter on the deck of the Titanic to save a few dollars.

Once the tests confirm your diagnosis, the third major step is to:

(3) *__Establish an antibiotic protocol__* that aggressively treats your condition. This is likely to be a combination of powerful antibiotics best suited for your condition and symptoms. Typically antibiotics treatment is augmented with one, or combinations, of the many drugs that the typical Lymer will already have been prescribed, including anti-depressants for depression; benzopaiedines such as Lorazepam, Clonazepam or Zanax for anxiety; Adderal or Ritalin for fatigue, concentration or attention deficits; and preferably the non-narcotic Lyrica (in lieu of dependency-forming narcotics like Vicodin or Oxycontin) for pain.

Once you and your doctor have established this, the fourth and final step is:

(4) *__Duration of treatment__*. A good LLMD (who is associated with ILADS) will be determined to see you to the finish line, for ***as long as it takes.*** For the critically ill who have been misdiagnosed for many months or years, this will require the same to undo the damage caused by treating the wrong disease. The corollary to number four here is **once you start treatment, *don't stop*.** Your best chance of beating this plague is to go the distance with no breaks or vacations. No shortcuts, miracle cures or quick fixes exist at this time; there are no silver bullets. Beware the many distractions and once under way, ***stay the course.***

Find a good LLMD, get tested at IGeneX, establish an antibiotic protocol that works, and stick with it until the bitter end. This is your best chance to get your life back.

Sounds easy? It could very well be the hardest journey of your life, but consider the alternative. Once you start, don't look back, and keep going until you have reached the Promised Land.

The Perplexing Tendency to "Avoid Treatment"

Astonishingly, some Lyme patients will do anything and everything under the sun to avoid getting tested or obtain treatment. A person afflicted with advanced late-stage Lyme is often unlikely to get the help they need on their own. The "artful dodger" comes to mind, like trying to corner a stray cat. The gradual onset of the disease can at first impair judgment, reason and the will, rendering the afflicted unable to act effectively on their own behalf. As perplexing as this sounds, it is not uncommon, and has been observed also amongst cancer patients and others with chronic or terminal diseases. As the first and most important of the four steps to a cure is to find a Lyme-literate doctor, or LLMD, this is often done by a concerned family member or close friend. After ten misdiagnoses over thirty-five years, and testing for Lyme for the third time before finding the right doctor with the right diagnosis, it took another person to intervene on my behalf to make this happen. That person was my mother, Jean Currier Amsden. With me at the time I was forty-nine years old!

The role of the Advocate, the Caretaker, and the Benefactor in the recovery of a Lyme victim is obviously advantageous in doing what it takes to get them the right help. A friend, family member or a loved one often assume this role, sometimes more than one or all three roles, and is likely essential for the support needed during the recovery period. Should it become necessary that you need help getting help, approach someone you can trust to get you where you need to be. As in my case and in the case of many others, reliance on family members and friends during the many months of antibiotic treatment are critical, as even the most basic tasks can be impossible.

Patience, persistence and sheer determination are essential during treatment. After establishing an antibiotic protocol that is effective, maintaining a persistent and consistent course for the duration, for as long as it takes, is essential to being cured. A stubborn countenance is helpful in these circumstances. It will test your resolve, your endurance, and your will.

In my case, it took 400mg of Biaxin, 200mg of Plaquenil, and 400mg of Doxycycline twice daily for forty-four (44) months before the symptoms finally subsided and recall only one time when the daily dose was forgotten—New Year's Eve 2010. And that was only for twelve hours! Though it was difficult, if not impossible, on most days to even tie my own shoes, the one thing, the *only* thing that really mattered was taking that daily protocol regularly and consistently.

That determination and consistency got me through to the end.

The role of "supplements"—diet, vitamins, natural herbs, and pharmaceuticals—all play an important role in your ability to withstand the excruciating symptoms of recovery. Medication to control pain, anxiety and depression are often essential. They are our "temporary friends" while we endure the course of treatment.

In my case, it was *Lyrica* for widespread pain, *Clonazepam* for severe anxiety and sleeplessness, *Prozac* for depression, *Amitriptyline* for dysautonomia, and *Adderal* for chronic fatigue, ADHD and the other post-traumatic stress disorder symptoms. These were absolutely necessary to withstand the relentless and excruciating symptoms of treatment. There were many times these temporary helpers were resisted, but in retrospect it was always at the expense of unnecessary and avoidable agony. There is *no advantage* to being resistant to taking these supplements—they are necessary, but temporary.

Now at the finish line, I am completely free of *all* these medications, including the antibiotics.

For most, money is an issue with Lyme treatment, even if you have more money than most. Health insurance, of course, like most doctors, do not recognize Lyme as a legitimate disease, and those resources are not generally available. In losing jobs, real estate, and essentially the ability to earn a living, the costs can be enormous, not to mention expensive doctor visits and medication. It could be questioned: "Is it worth the risk to lose everything?" But consider the alternative. There is no cost too great to have one's life back.

Health before wealth.

Often this occurs by prevailing on Social Security Disability Income (SSDI.) Applying based upon one or more of the many options available in the myriad of manifestations the disease can take, consider these options:

- Multiple Sclerosis
- Parkinson's' disease
- Bi-polar Disease
- Chronic Fatigue Syndrome
- Schizophrenia
- Alzheimer's
- ADD, ADHD, PTSD
- Dysautonomia
- ALS
- Lupus
- Rheumatoid arthritis
- Dementia
- Fibromyalgia
- Obsessive-Compulsive Disorder (OCD)
- Depression
- Autism
- Asperger's Syndrome

And the list goes on. Most likely you will find yourself in one or more of these categories if you have Lyme. Once obtained, disability benefits will cover many of the associated costs of treatment, even though Lyme treatment is not recognized or covered. The alternative of a nursing home, hospice, and in the end, death are not the desired outcomes.

No matter what it costs, and what sacrifices must be made, a life worth living is one that is based upon good health.

When it comes down to paying the mortgage, the credit cards, or the car payment—compared to getting better—there is no alternative. You will need to do what needs to be done. *Period.*

And, a final remark about plain old-fashioned dumb luck. In my case, it was fortunate indeed that the right conditions were in place. To have my mother intervene on my behalf and setup that third test with a Lyme-literate doctor—there are many reasons why this may have never occurred. To have a Benefactor who understands and who can afford to support you, a Caretaker who understands and is willing to care for the daily needs; sometimes you just have to be lucky. I am one of the lucky ones. In fact, I am the luckiest person, by far, that I have ever known.

2014: The Lymester On-line Advocacy

Organized on July 22nd, 2014, "*The Lymester*" began its debut on YouTube as a Lyme-advocacy site to share these experiences and to foster ongoing discussion and awareness. The trials and tribulations experienced by the Lyme victim, our failures and successes, are now available to those who seek information and knowledge and perhaps to take comfort in knowing they are not alone, that others are experiencing the same or similar ordeals. But most importantly, that the ordeal can be overcome, that there does exist a road to victory that has been achieved by others.

And there does exist a cure.

But advocating for others sometimes reveals disturbing patterns of willful self-destruction. Reaching back to rescue my youngest daughter, even while I was still in recovery, taught me several things about advocating for others. One, you can really only save the ones you love; and two, only those who actually *want* to get well *will* get well. This second realization is still the hardest to accept. Who could possibly not want to escape the agony of this debacle? But over and over while advocating personally for other Lyme victims, a recurring pattern persisted among some to resist diagnosis and treatment, even when the path to victory seemed clear. For these patients, self-sabotage or subterfuge would seem unlikely given the circumstances, but clearly illustrates an astonishing self-denial when it comes to treatment. A self-deprecating sense of *deserving* extreme suffering becomes self-inflicted. Knowing that the root of much, if not most, of psychiatric illness in modern society has its origin in the Lyme spirochete or related infectious diseases does little for the sufferer. There is a sense of inescapable fate that seizes some Lyme victims. Accepted with resignation, acquiescing to powers seemingly beyond one's control, destruction of the faculties of reason and will take a heavy toll.

Including the will to live.

The Lymester advocacy provides many opportunities to further research, not only the nature of the disease and its many manifestations, but also the very nature of suffering itself.

Uncovering the tendency of some to avoid treatment, even to the point of violently defending their right to deny it, shed light on a mysterious condition beyond just Lyme. Why would anyone choose to accept suffering, even seemingly *demand* it, in the face of possible cure? Why do some seem to willingly embrace hopelessness for reasons unknown to the victim or the observer? This most perplexing condition led to many hours of further research and contemplation. Mysterious as it seems, there are some who seem absolutely determined to ensure the continuation of their own suffering, even when presented the real possibility of reversing their condition.

At first, I had great difficulty with accepting this. The advocacy continued relentlessly to admonish victims who would do nothing to help themselves. I found myself often pleading with those who would do anything and everything under the sun, *except* the one thing that would actually help them. These examples of self-destructive behavior were more frequent than might be expected. It seemed these victims, by their own hand, are their own worst enemy when it comes to getting well again. Self-subterfuge was there at every step, to dissuade, derail, disconnect, and dis-continue any progress toward recovery. It was beyond reason. Irrational choices made again and again in the face of deepening despair and declining health were actually *demanded* (and often militantly defended) over obvious common-sense alternatives that would have ensured recovery. Over and over this mysterious phenomena would prevail on the afflicted who struggled with *and* defended it at the same time.

After much soul-searching on this issue, and further research and intensive study, it became clear that there was something more going on here than just Lyme. It occurred to me that there is a diabolical side to the issue of Lyme on a much larger scale, beyond the scope of Lyme, of disease, and of human suffering in general. It seemed that human suffering and its origins played a much larger role in the victims of Lyme than just the Borrelia spirochete. There are some surprising conclusions drawn from this research in tracing back the root of human suffering to its origins, of which few are prepared and even fewer willing to know or accept.

We have become comfortable in our ignorance and taught to deny those aspects of our daily lives that would otherwise disrupt our comfort zone.

As observed in the complications of the current Lyme plague, we see the same conditions nurtured by the seeds of misery and denial, and finally flourishing in decline and decay. As in all past plagues, rooted by degree in the higher realms of our spirituality or lack thereof, we create for ourselves the very conditions that are reflected back upon on us by nature. These are of necessity manifested and guided by the universal laws of nature, and their influence upon the human spirit is self-generated.

My own path is testimony to this. The *Lymester* advocacy, devoted to documenting this journey, emphasizes that by whatever light shines upon this path to well-being might become a beacon for those who choose to find their way. It is by this tradition of holding the light aloft that others who seek it may find their way "home" again.

The Psychiatric Manifestations of Lyme Disease

Oct. 4, 2014: Most people still remain unaware of the many psychiatric manifestations of Lyme disease. Usually the early symptoms are attributed to one or more of the numerous disorders of the mind, often displayed at first mildly in behavioral issues in adults and more recently and in greater frequency in children. Both neurological and/or psychological, these frequently fall into these categories:

- Attention Deficit Disorder (ADD)
- Attention Deficit Hyperactive Disorder (ADHD)
- Obsessive Compulsive Disorder (OCD)
- Epilepsy
- Autism Spectrum Disorder
- Asperger's syndrome
- Anxiety disorders
- Anger or uncontrolled rage issues

There is increasing evidence suggesting that the prevalence of autism among infants could be a result of misdiagnosis. Often attributed to unexplained learning disabilities, mental impairment, and environmental-behavioral factors, it is possible that these children, born of mother's who are unknowingly infected with Borrelia, or possibly related sources such as mycoplasma—which has been discovered in vaccines—may instead have Lyme. Traditional views of heredity disease due to genetic causes are slowly yielding to this new data, as this could easily be misinterpreted as such. Typically, the source of these conditions is never identified, nor are they even sought by the family physician. All too eager to prescribe pharmaceutical "solutions" designed only to suppress the worse of the symptoms, the underlying cause remains to flourish in favor of placating the effects and covering up the facts. This is a perfect model for generating profits.

Could the Lyme spirochete Borrelia and the myriad of co-infections be the root of many forms of "mental illness" that plague our society?

Continuing undetected, the actual cause of affliction continues to manifest in increasing severity, and morphs into other more serious conditions, often misdiagnosed as:

- Depression
- Bi-polar Disorder
- Schizophrenia
- Borderline Personality Disorder
- Post-Traumatic Stress Disorder (PTSD)
- Chronic Anxiety Disorder
- Chronic Fatigue Syndrome
- Nymphomania
- Fibromyalgia
- Hypochondria
- Psychopathy
- Socio-pathology
- Narcissism
- Sadomasochism
- Necrophilia

Adolescents who develop depression or bi-polar issues can progress to other more debilitating conditions such as personality disorders, psychopathy, schizophrenia, narcissism, and socio-pathology, with the consequences of bullying, teenage suicide, and sexually deviant behavior. As the age group for these individuals advances in years, the tendency to label these as psychopaths, sociopaths, schizophrenics, hypochondriacs, or as "malingerers" as adults is a most common reaction amongst psychiatrists. Attributing symptoms as a manifestation of psychosis, a figment of imagination, need for attention, or other maladjusted behavior fits their narrow definition for treatment of symptoms with pharmaceutical therapy. As is the case for all age groups, the root causes of these early symptoms are dismissed or ignored in favor of placating the symptoms with numerous mind-altering drugs.

It is not difficult to understand the financial incentive for a doctor to treat a disease rather than cure it. It is the same pattern of ignoring the root causes in favor of treatment of symptoms by prescription that can be found in *all* areas of medicine. This prolongs the misdiagnosis, causing the disease to further manifest while the patient suffers increasing debilitation. This, in turn, creates an artificial demand for further treatment at increasingly higher cost. The caveat here is that while these symptom-abating methods can be helpful or even necessary in alleviating the symptoms *while you are being cured*, they are not an end in itself.

The social and economic consequences of this are enormous. In recent years, the episodes of horrific violence by those who were later discovered to be afflicted in the brain with advanced Lyme borreliosis are a small example of the high cost to society for ignoring this problem. "Lyme-rage" is a common symptom of the severely compromised Lyme victim, where the spread of the disease causes inflammation in brain tissue associated with the neocortex and other parts of the brain. In his book "*The Anatomy of Human Self-Destruction*" (1973), Erich Fromm states from the standpoint of neuroscience how the brain can become the basis for aggressive behavior learned through environmental based character passions:

> *"Given the dual organization of the brain, the crucial question arises: What are the factors that disturb the balance and produce manifest rage and corresponding violent behavior? We have already seen that one way in which such disturbance of the balance can be produced is by electric stimulation or destruction of any inhibitory areas (aside from hormonal and metabolic changes)... [these] emphasize that such disturbance of the equilibrium can also occur due to various forms of <u>brain disease that alter the normal circuity of the brain</u>. But what are the conditions that change the equilibrium and mobilize aggression,*

aside from these two instances, one of which is experimentally introduced and the other pathological? What are the causes of 'innate' aggression in animals and humans?"

What are the causes, indeed! We see the same pattern repeated over and over in Lyme patient symptoms of severe chronic fatigue on one hand, and the exaggerated "fight or flight" syndrome or Post Traumatic Stress Disorder (PTSD) and Lyme-rage on the other. Could this maladaptive form of aggression be explained by disease or inflammation of the brain from the Lyme borrelia spirochete? Meanwhile, the real problem deliberately ignored, treatment for chronic Lyme conditions continue to be systemically denied. In direct violation of the Hippocratic Oath that all doctors, by law and by ethical standards, are sworn to uphold, we are taught to believe that no doctor would ever knowingly or willingly cause harm to a patient. Prevailing wisdom, however, suggests this simply is not the case.

Beware the narrative of the family doctor, psychiatrist or psychologist who insist that it is "all in your head."

This may be technically correct, but misleading as to its actual cause. The effects of the Lyme spirochete are known to parallel syphilis on the human brain, and many documented cases of dementia and related symptoms can be cited. Inflammation and destruction of brain tissue are well known as root causes of behavioral and physical disorders, and as Fromm has stated, cultivate fertile ground for character-based flaws that involve behavioral, personality and identity issues. Given the widespread nature of the stealthy dissemination of Lyme, there exists a high probability as the origin or source of the significant rise in these modern-day afflictions. To ignore this possibility, with what we know after forty years or more of becoming acquainted with the Lyme spirochete, it is at best a tragedy of epidemic proportions.

Due to negligent malpractice, and at worse, *intentional, willful negligence* on the part of the medical community, the deliberate attempts to deny, hide, mislead and suppress this information has become the "lie too big to admit." Doing otherwise would expose the doctors, researchers and administrators to a liability so great that it could only be classified as criminal. Meanwhile, the silent epidemic continues across the nation and around the globe.

A "Family Affair"

1985-2015: Preceded by my aunt, who was diagnosed with multiple sclerosis during the mid-1980's, youngest daughter Leah was the first in our family to be diagnosed with Lyme in the early 1990's, when she was five years old. Little did we know then that I would be next, some twenty years later, followed by my father—with babesiosis—and my younger brother, Randall, soon after. By then, the disease had manifested in each of us, taking its toll as it ever so slowly debilitated the body and mind, one cell at a time, gradually, stealthily and barely perceptible. Again, the "boiling frog" metaphor comes to mind, where the frog in the pot, when heated slowly, is unaware that it is being boiled until it is too late to get out.

In my case, several decades went by before I gradually succumbed to the affliction and was diagnosed. My dad, on the other hand, was diagnosed immediately after an acute bout with babesia in the mid-2000's. However, my youngest brother also went about 20+ years before being diagnosed, as did my youngest daughter. None of us were aware that the slight disturbances slowly evolving in our physical health could be attributed to Lyme, despite our personal and sometimes heroic efforts to fend off its advances. We were all land surveyors, having followed my dad in the business of hacking trails through the woods to peer between the leaves and branches with a transit in the coarser art of map making. Heat, insects, poison ivy and pucker-brush were all part of the game, and we were well-suited for and experienced in daily adversity of these types. Many times, we recall pulling ticks off of our clothes and out of the skin, as would anyone who finds themselves, even for brief periods, hiking, hunting or camping in the New England woods.

In the late 1990's and early 2000's, it seemed that the tick population had exploded in New Hampshire, Massachusetts, Maine and Vermont, and was steadily spreading in all directions, especially south and west. Attributed to rising deer populations, this continues through the present day. In fact, ticks are threatening the local moose population. At the current rate, extinction is predicted by year 2045. Dead moose have been found literally drained of blood by over 100,000 ticks attached to them.

More reports and warnings of the spread of Lyme are seen in the local daily newspapers, but suspiciously little from the medical community or the larger cable news networks, asleep at the wheel or in a seemingly self-induced coma about the spreading epidemic. Their silence has become a deafening roar to the afflicted, as increasingly there are local reports of strange disorders appearing in clusters within certain areas throughout the northeast, the Midwest, and the furthest reaches of the west. This is no longer a rare occurrence, and with escalating frequency we hear of pockets of communities stricken by a mysterious illness, and somehow the medical community cannot see, or come to terms with, what is so obviously right in front of their face. Pressured for quick answers, a rush to judgment usually results in arriving at some phony diagnosis.

It is a shameful affair during this time of technological progress that here in the 21st century modern medicine has handled this epidemic.

Concentration and focus on proliferation of disease and its profits over cures and affordable health-care foretells our current ordeal today. As a result, the tendency in modern medicine favors a *cult of deception and diversion.* Emergence of the evidence will eventually surface and is already beginning to set the record straight.

EXCLUSIVE INTERVIEW: Leah (Amsden) Fontane

Feb, 2nd, 2015: After twenty-three years of struggling with the disease since childhood, Leah Amsden-Fontane describes her ordeal in a powerful narrative about growing up with Lyme disease in Concord, New Hampshire. As a young child, teenager and into adulthood, here described are the extraordinary circumstances and effort it took to overcome it. Surely an inspirational testament of hope for those in despair, it is testimony that there are treatments that work, that a cure exists, and that there is real hope for a normal life again.

Leah first exhibited symptoms after her family returned from camping near Enfield, Connecticut, in 1990 when she was just five years old. This quaint old New England town is only miles from "ground zero" in Lyme, Connecticut, where the first cases of Lyme were detected some twenty years earlier. (This is where the name "Lyme" originated.) Frequent common illnesses such as colds, unusual rashes, and minor behavioral or cognitive impairments started to appear, until finally one day in tears, she complained about extreme pain in her knees, making it difficult for her to walk. Perplexed, the family physician recommended an orthopedic specialist who ran a series of blood tests. Her father insisted on a Lyme test against the advice of the orthopedic doctor, who at first refused but at the insistence of the father, reluctantly, approved the test.

His prognosis: "*juvenile arthritis*."

Naproxyn was prescribed, and little else was forthcoming until six months later while returning to a new family physician, who upon reading her charts exclaimed, "So, how is Leah being treated for Lyme?" Completely caught off guard, her father gasped and replied, "What do you mean *Lyme*?" The doctor replied, "Her blood test shows the Lyme-titer as positive for Lyme." The earlier orthopedic specialist, who had displayed such arrogance in first refusing the test for Lyme six months earlier, had never even bothered to look at the results when he served his predetermined sentence of "juvenile arthritis." Meanwhile, because of the naproxyn, which dilates the blood vessels, the disease had further manifested—undetected—for over six months, all throughout her body.

I'll never forget that day, as I am Leah's father.

The new family doctor immediately admitted her, that same day, to the hospital for three days of IV treatment with the powerful Ceftriaxone antibiotic and continued the IV treatment at home for the next thirty days. With a port in her arm, she endured the horrific treatment that comes with the excruciating "herx" reactions. An in-home nurse came each week to change the port, which, needless to say, is a very traumatic experience for a five-year-old. Holding her down while she screamed in anguish was traumatic for her parents as well, as the enormity of what had happened.

This was deeply disturbing, to say the least. No effort was made on the part of this doctor to acknowledge anything, and insurance attorneys representing the practice were invoked. Obviously, they were fearful of repercussions, and that seemed to be all that concerned them. That their patient suffered as a result of their negligence was never acknowledged or corrected.

As the hero of the story, Leah's new family doctor acted aggressively admitting her to the emergency room for IV treatment for 72 hours, followed by rigorous home IV therapy for another thirty days with Ceftriaxone. Though unconvinced himself that she had been fully cured, he made repeated attempts to reassure her parents about the controversy of short-term antibiotic treatment being enough to eradicate the spirochete completely. At the time, this prognosis was reluctantly accepted, as the doctor had a look in his eye of uncertainty that betrayed his words of reassurance. During continued care for Leah throughout her growing years into adolescence and early adulthood, he would often prescribe antibiotics for the many symptoms and conditions that emerged as a result. For every cold, rash or fever, he would consistently prescribe up to two weeks of antibiotics.

Deepest intuition told me that this doctor maintained a persistent doubt in the back of his mind of the purported "cure" justified in the medical journals about Lyme. At that time, much less was known about the disease, and his actions exposed this doubt. Often it occurred to me that he was reassuring *us* that she was cured but continued to treat her based upon real doubt about the prevailing belief in the efficacy of "short-term treatment" and that Lyme was easy to cure. Certainly what was to come confirmed his suspicion, as experience is our best teacher.

In the years that followed, Leah's advancement through elementary school, junior high and emerging as a young adult were far from "normal" in the sense of overall general health and particularly in behavior. She exhibited symptoms of OCD (obsessive compulsive disorder), not being able to "let things go," and would go "on and on" at times about not getting her way.

Though not in itself unusual for a child her age, it was the *extreme nature* of it that stood out. She had difficulties with socialization and suffered a rather severe identity crisis at a crucial time in the development of personality. For her parents, the underlying notion that things were not right was confirmed by another specialist who determined frontal lobe damage to the brain could be the cause of these anomalies— damage believed to be from the previous Lyme infection, which it was presumed at the time had been cured.

Her parents carried on with the grim reality that Lyme disease had permanently debilitated their daughter, and with great difficulty struggled with the fact that the original test was positive and had gone undetected by the attending doctor. Possible legal action was considered, and a meeting with the insurance company was scheduled. The insurance company took the typical defensive position with no acknowledgement of negligence or wrongdoing, and the parents backed down in futility by what appeared to be no way of recourse. We learned the hard way why Lyme is not considered a legitimate condition.

Meanwhile, Leah continued to struggle in school, her studies suffered, as did her social life in adjusting to a world with others that was taking place as if behind a glass wall. She would often become obsessed with Disney movies that she watched over and over to live in a fantasy world that she increasingly was unable to emerge from. Her emotional reactions to everyday life were extreme. The typical whack-a-mole approach to ongoing treatment had Leah's ship on stormy waters. The more she tried to cope with persistent effects believed at the time a permanent disability, the more psychiatric medication was prescribed and the further the disease was permitted to advance.

Her first "true love" experience in junior high led to anxiety and vomiting as a reaction to the emotional strain, and her father feared bulimia or anorexia as a possible new development. The normal kind of agonies experienced by a typical teenager were larger than life itself for Leah, as she struggled to keep the pendulum of her experiences from swinging too wildly out of control. The ability to internally balance the experiences of growing up were often too much to handle and would manifest in the extremes of behavioral excesses or deficits such as Attention Deficit Disorder (ADD), Attention Deficit Hyperactive Disorder (ADHD), Obsessive Compulsive Disorder (OCD).

Leah was especially sensitive to the excruciating self-awareness of not being quite right, and the sense that she was somehow different and/or maladjusted. This further exacerbated the cycle of self-identity problems she fought vigorously against, the tidal forces that continuously threatened her fragile identity. Her courageous struggle against unseen forces beyond her control were heroic for one so young who since five years old had not been given a fair shake at life. High school proved her struggle would be sometimes overcome, as in art and music she exemplified great prowess and ability against indescribable odds, and her grades at times would rise above the average and even soar during the ebb and flow of her affliction. This revealed a tremendous potential under the rough exterior of troubles she endured, and as she went on to college and experienced otherwise normal relationships, she proved again and again that she could achieve her dreams even with the demons that continued to plague and interfere with these efforts. Her marriage and beginnings in working careers further exemplified her ability to overcome and carry on. That is, until around year 2012, after two years of marriage with her new husband, Victor Fontane, she began a series of downward spirals in emotional quagmires that threatened the fragile balance she had achieved.

Meanwhile, by year 2010, I also was finally diagnosed with Lyme and at last understood the cause of my long demise and that I, too, was slowly suffering the same fate. Loss of the ability to work, foreclosure, bankruptcy and divorce. Finally destitute, my disability attorney assured me that I had a 95% chance of securing my financial future once again through SSDI (Social Security Disability Income), and the arduous return to life began with treatment that proved more harsh than the journey yet endured.

Lyme is a doubly cruel disease for those fortunate enough to discover that they have it, find a doctor who will treat them, can afford to pay for it when insurance abandons them, and endure the severity of long-term treatment. After finally prevailing with Social Security Disability and two years into treatment, 95% debilitated, crippled and completely disabled, by 2012 I noticed Leah was having extreme difficulty with anxiety disorders that threatened their young marriage and her ability to cope with everyday life. The idea of returning to her orthodox Jewish heritage beckoned as a form of sanctuary from the chaos of the outside world. I instinctively knew without question the original source and cause of her downward spiral, and memory of all her past struggles and tribulations came flooding back in an overwhelming urgency to act quickly.

I knew, without a doubt, that Leah's Lyme disease from her childhood had not in fact ever been cured. Despite the level of delirium and daily torture endured in my own treatment, I knew the timing of Leah's rescue was reaching a critical moment, and I swiftly intervened as only a father can and grabbed the rudder of her unsteady ship.

Upon my insistence, Leah and husband Victor agreed to see a prominent Lyme-literate doctor nearby in Washington, DC. The doctor was very receptive to her condition and history, and subsequent test results from IGeneX proved positive for Lyme antibodies. The doctor immediately started her on a powerful antibiotic protocol combination that generated the typical "herx" dementia that is so difficult to endure. This further emphasized that after all those long years of her early life, the original 30-day IV treatment that supposedly had "cured" her of Lyme had been completely ineffective in ridding her body of the spirochete, which continued to manifest over the next two decades of her life.

Several things about this crucial event are in retrospect *miraculous.*

Succumbing to my own fate just months before brought a new understanding of the disease, and the critical importance of long-term antibiotic treatment as the surest way to recovery and cure. Secondly, even after two decades of suffering, Leah had not yet reached the point of no return, where hopelessness succumbs to *refusing to get well.*

This simply cannot be overemphasized.

The following chapter on the *Affliction of The Spirit: The Diabolical Side of Lyme Disease* further discusses the way in which the disease not only "switches off" or disables the immune system, but renders the faculties of reason, desire and will as inoperable, and can turn the Lyme victim against themselves in a most illogical, subterfugical and self-destructive way. It can literally destroy the will to survive. The fact that Leah still had the will and the *desire* to get well, that she desperately *wanted* to get her life back, were critical elements in the timing of her rescue. She did not refuse getting tested or resist the idea of treatment, which were absolutely necessary for the turnaround of events to come. Sometimes it is difficult to determine precisely when these turns of events occur, but not in this instance. Imploring her on the phone to see a Lyme-literate doctor who would determine, once and for all, whether the source of her affliction was the old Lyme from he early 1990's, she agreed. And at that very second, her ship was steered in a new direction; the direction home to the Promised Land.

In her own words:

Exclusive Interview with Leah Fontane (Transcript)

"How I Was CURED from Lyme Disease"

From YouTube Channel:

The Lymester

Published on Feb 2, 2015

"There's more than one way to see the impact of Lyme awareness, and one is on a singular level, and it's my own, and being interviewed, and really formally thinking back on my past and knowing my story and what I went through knowing where I am now, that is it meets the satisfactory aspect of my life just to really understand the whole of things. And on a broader level, my story brings awareness to others so if people can understand what I've been through, and what I call a more unusual case of Lyme disease, then it's good for them, but it's also good for me to kind of see it from a different perspective, because I've only seen it through my own eyes, almost like tunnel vision. This is my life, this is my experience, this is what I feel, this is what I go through whereas if I talk about it like I'm trying to explain myself to others, I actually can see it more from their perspective, and how they may see me. So, help me learn more about myself.

I was born in Columbia, Maryland and then I moved up to New Hampshire when I was about three. I was raised there for most of my youth until I graduated high school.

Question: So, how old were you when you were first bitten by a tick, what year was it, if you recall?

When I was actually about, I was probably three, maybe just barely four.

Question: What year would you say?

That would have been 1988-1989?

Question: Where location-wise were you bitten?

If I remember correctly, I believe my parents said that I was bitten on a camping trip in Connecticut. It may have been New Hampshire, but I believe it was Connecticut.

Question: At about that time did you guys know that you had Lyme, or did it take a while to see symptoms and then figure it?

Nobody was aware I had Lyme when I first picked it up. For a year people were not aware that I had Lyme. I started getting arthritis pains and some flu symptoms, and I got diagnosed with rheumatoid arthritis - juvenile rheumatoid arthritis - and they treated me for that for about a year. And if I remember correctly, I did get tested, and they found later that it actually even showed on my early blood tests that I had Lyme disease, but it wasn't even discussed until a year later during a routine follow-up visit with my doctor. I remember my mom standing in the hall by the pharmacy with my doctor, and my doctor just looked at my mom and said, "How's her treatment for Lyme was going?" My mom's eyes got really big as she's like—what? I don't know the full story on how; it is kind of like it was documented but we weren't aware of it. It got overlooked somehow, for a year. Yes, I got misdiagnosed with this really unusual disease. It's very uncommon for children to have arthritis, but it's easier to believe that I have this really unusual disease then the possibility that these symptoms might actually be something more common like Lyme disease. At least that's how it was at that time.

Question: So, once you discovered it, or your parents discovered, that you had Lyme disease, did you get treated for it?

Yes, I did. I remember the day I arrived at the hospital. I actually got to ride in a wheelchair, and not only was that kind of cool in this big fancy hospital, to be wheeled in a chair, but also at that moment I remember feeling sick, and feeling scared for so long. And not that people didn't take it seriously, I mean, I was still being treated for an illness, but when they sat me down in that wheelchair, I don't know if the nurse said something to explain why or if it was just something I internalized at that moment, but I literally felt a sense of relief, like the wheelchair represented the truth, and that it was a reality, that there was really something wrong with me. It's kind of like I got to let it go and just surrender to the wheelchair. Whereas I do remember my parents trying to have me keep up when we were like on hiking trips so that I did not stay too stuck on my "arthritis." I don't know how clear those memories are, but I do remember the feeling of the wheelchair being a sense of relief and surrender.

Question: You knew then you were going to be taken care of?

Yes, yes, you got it, I knew at that moment I was being taken care of in the way that really suited how I really felt, which was sick.

Question: How long were you treated for?

It was, I think I was in the hospital for four days, and the entire treatment process was about three weeks, maybe there's like a follow-up appointment. And I remember my mom saying that even after I was fully treated and I had my checkup and I was good to go, the doctor still like gave one more dose of medicine to my parents and said something like "just in case."

Question: So, about three weeks of antibiotics?

Yes, three weeks of antibiotics, and when I was in the hospital I had IV antibiotics. And I remember having the IV for at least a little while once I came home actually, wheeling it around in the house.

Question: It must have been difficult for your parents, their child attached to an IV like that?

I think the whole experience was probably more traumatizing for my parents than it probably was for me, and it was pretty scary for me, too.

Question: So, after three weeks, did the treatment work?

Well, now that we understand how it all works, yes, it did help at the moment. I went into the hospital with severe pain in my joints and feeling very fatigued, and flu symptoms, common flu symptoms, and when I left, and when I was treated until the end, I remember the pain went away. I felt better. But it wasn't the end of it. It was sort of short-lived.

Question: What symptoms did linger?

It was hard to remember exactly which symptoms were immediately still apparent at that age, and I was going on five into kindergarten, but I remember feeling uptight, anxious, even scared, but really more realistically, I was tense. I remember I just never felt right. I always felt kind of agitated and like I couldn't contain my energy, and I also remember feeling sick to my stomach, nauseous. I even remember learning what the word *anxious* meant because I used to complain frequently that I was nauseous. Eventually I had a psychological evaluation, and they diagnosed me with anxiety. I was five, but a five-year-old child that hasn't gone through like severe trauma, yeah I mean, I had my couple of days in the hospital, but still I wasn't abused or raped, didn't witness somebody dying or violence or anything like that. So, I had a couple days in the hospital, but I had *severe* anxiety, and so I learned the difference between nausea and anxiety, but really when I look back on it, it was all kind of the same. It's just the more anxious, the more nauseous I would get. I would get car sick often and remember waking up in the middle of the night a lot also having trouble falling asleep. And then of course in early school I had trouble learning. That was I think the biggest giveaway, that there was still something wrong, not to say that learning disabilities don't exist, of course they do, but, it just didn't add up, didn't make sense. In some ways I was very bright, but in other ways when it came to the more technical aspect of learning, I struggled.

Question: So, you had issues at school?

Sure, I definitely had issues at school. I remember doing this special education piece of the class, having a teacher's aide actually work with me to help me learn how to read. But what I do distinctly remember is the day that I passed my exam. It was sort of an exam for children where I didn't have to do the reading class anymore. I did it very well; I was congratulated and honored like I did such a good job. So, if I was able to eventually learn how to do it, it means that I always had the ability to do it. I just remember always feeling uncomfortable, like I was tense and uptight, and I couldn't sit still. It wasn't that my brain didn't work, it was that there was something funky going on inside of my body, and it was to the point where I was too distracted to sit still and pay attention, to really focus on something. I had to be very motivated, which is why that special education class helped me.

Question: Did you continue to have these struggles throughout elementary school, middle school, high school, and did you go back to any treatment during your school years?

Well, when I was growing up, I already talked about how I struggled as a very a young child learning how to read and to focus in school, but it lasted with me through all of my schooling years, through the rest of elementary school, middle school, high school. I would say that I struggled most in school in my adolescent years, especially the middle school age.

No, I never received any more treatment for Lyme disease. With all of these other struggles that I had growing up, I was misdiagnosed and treated for all those other "disorders." Lyme disease was never even considered. I was treated. I did my three weeks of antibiotics. I should be good, so whatever I've got now still bothering me, whatever I'm still struggling with, that must have just been other problems. Right?

Question: Psychological problems?

Oh yeah, psychological. I know it was, I remember. I believe I was six or seven when I was diagnosed with obsessive-compulsive disorder. Let me repeat that, *obsessive-compulsive disorder*. For a first grader? What could be so complex about the life of a six or seven-year-old that would make it so that they'd be obsessive compulsive? But I didn't have the same key obsessive-compulsive behaviors like obsessively washing hands, or having irrational fears, and getting stuck on them and not being able to move on, and it being debilitating. I didn't have that. I just I would get stuck on things that I wanted, or if I get upset, I'd get *really* upset, or some would say I overreacted, but it wasn't classic obsessive-compulsive disorder. Again, something just wasn't right. Something was missing. Didn't add up. And then I also remember, by the time I was about seven or eight I was already taking Ritalin. And then I believe the next medicine they added to the mix was Clonidine, which helped with anxiety and depression. So, obsessive-compulsive disorder, ADHD and anxiety, I think I had all of those disorders by the age of nine or ten. So, by upper elementary school and through middle school into high school,

I was being medicated for multiple disorders; not just one, several.

Question: Most of the medicines that you were taking throughout your school years were psychological and/or psychiatric medicines for the most part?

Yes, so I think all of the medicines that I was taking throughout my youth were for psychological disorders, a concoction of medicines, not even just one to take care of it all; it was more than one. And, I was medicated throughout my whole youth.

Question: So, it seems that living with Lyme really impaired your lifestyle and impaired what you were capable of. How were you able to cope with that?

I don't think I coped all that much to be honest. I was expressive in arts. I did music, art and theater. I didn't really get into all that until I was really an adolescent. But I do remember I spent quite a bit of time playing on the piano, and then I started to learn how to sing and started even writing my own songs, and it was really the only outlet that I had for all of the energy that seemed to always be just pent up inside with nowhere to go. And I would go to school and enjoy being in the class with others, but always struggled to pay attention, always struggled to study and to do my work, but when I would come home, I would go right to my music or doing a piece of art or enjoying nature. It was a way for me to shut off my mind. In other words, really not have to use it, and even though I always felt uncomfortable inside, when it didn't require that I focused on anything intently that required mental focus, brain activity, it was a lot easier. I was able to forget about the discomfort and just be, whereas doing real intellectual thought, intellectual work, like in class, it really required that I just sit there. I wasn't allowed to move. I had to stay in one spot, I had to stare at a book for long periods of time, or I had to write, and I remember being almost excruciatingly uncomfortable. To just sit felt like I had a very subtle electrical current running through my body, like my blood had something that responded to electricity, and it was just this constant field of energy flowing all in and around my body, especially in my chest area, and head, which is why it was like having severe anxiety. My nerves could not chill; and when anything would set me off, anytime my nerves were stimulated, I would go from a neutral state to a really high stress state in seconds. I remember when I would have the severe anxiety, and it would cause nausea and vomiting. I would go from being totally fine to something making me really nervous or frightening me. If it was like having to go to a doctor and have a shot, or just sometimes it was even just emotional stress, I would just skyrocket to this swell-up of adrenaline and nausea, and then I would vomit within two or three minutes. It would come on that fast, not like a flu where you get a little bit of a stomach ache and then you feel a little sicker, no, so this was like bada-boom bada-bing. Took no time at all.

I remember it happened when I got my ears pierced for my 10th birthday. It's like getting a shot in each ear. I even remember like, oh, that wasn't that bad, and then after they did the other ear, I had just been so worked up about it, so tense, so anxious, shaking, just anticipating it, that when it actually happened, the adrenaline went through my body, and within a couple of minutes I had to get sick in the trash can, right in the jewelry shop! I wasn't even really bothered by the actual piercing. It was quick. It was easy. But my body overreacted. It's kind of like my body did its own thing, whereas, no, I was really okay, but my body was not, and this was just something that I went through for years, years, and years. I've only very recently had relief from this condition, of just not being able to have control over my nerves, and there being no middle ground between being neutral and being very high-stress, like when people have really traumatic experiences that would really scare you. But simple things like getting my ears pierced or having to go to the doctors to get my blood taken, even going to a counseling office talking about myself, I just remembered being so anxious, I had to get sick. It wasn't a reason to get sick, again, it didn't add up. Something was wrong; something was missing.

Question: Did those struggles have any effect on your relationships with others?

Sure. I mean, I spent my whole childhood always feeling like there was something wrong with me, that my behavior was unacceptable. When I would be excited, I would be *very* excited. When I was angry, I would be *very* angry. And I also had a tendency to go on, on, on, and on. I couldn't stop it when I would be passionate about something, or I wanted something, or I was upset about something. I wouldn't just complain, I would go on and on and on and on and on and if I didn't feel like I was getting the direct attention, I would just keep pushing. And you know, this was always something that my parents implied was selfishness, and that wasn't really it – no, it wasn't directly said "this is not okay Leah," but I always felt like it wasn't okay for me to be stuck, for me to behave like that, for me to be so dramatic. But when your body is at a state of sensitivity, normal emotions trigger the same bodily response as extreme emotions, so again, there was no middle ground. If I was feeling an emotion, I was feeling it up here (over head). It was very hard for me to have a conversation about almost anything without getting overly dramatic, and usually eventually upset, because I remembered the adrenaline. The feeling was so awful. So, when I was mad about something, it felt so bad that I couldn't contain myself. I would become enraged. It's hard not to. Even when just frustrated, my body felt like I was enraged. It was like a switch just turned on, and there I go – there, I'm in that state again.

Question: These struggles also affect your personal relationships?

Oh ya, they did. I would say these struggles affected my relationship with my friends and my peers more than my family, because my family knew me, and even though they didn't know I had Lyme disease, they understood that I was a little "off." I was different, and they still loved me for it. I had unconditional love from my family, but with friendships, and with peers, it was different because people didn't know the whole me. And when I would be in school, even in class, I would be talking about something, if I felt nervous I might stutter, or I might say a word, might just get thrown in the middle of a sentence that doesn't belong there. Or a word that rhymes with the correct word is said but it's not the word I meant to say what happened, or you would just be able to tell that I felt befuddled, like I had marble-mouth. And the more nervous I was, the more it would affect my communication.

So, just in a normal social setting, if I was nervous, which is typical for a teenager to be nervous, I'm really sure it came across as strange at times. There were also times where I was just able to talk away and there was no problem at all, but there were of course other times where it was challenging. It's like my speech was challenged, like an impediment, and I think that I came across as maybe less intelligent than I really was. I was always such a bright and intelligent person. Always, I always knew it. I knew what was inside of me; I knew what my brain really was, always, but it was as if I was an exceptional, highly intellectual individual trapped inside a disabled body. And because I knew it, and because I wanted to be the person that I always knew I really was, then I would be in those situations where I would try to project myself as I am, who I really am, and it wouldn't come out the way that I really was. It was extremely frustrating, and I could see it. Like my peers may have had their own opinion about who I was, how I behaved, what it meant, why I acted that weird way, or why I said those weird things, or why I would be overly expressive, made funny faces, or why I was always so stressed, moving, always so nervous, always so insecure, so that's who I was in the eyes of others.

But I knew who I really was, and I knew that when that funky thing that was going on in my body wasn't happening, I was just like everybody else—I could carry on a perfectly normal conversation like I'm doing right now. But when I was in the situation where I needed to be at my best, I was usually at my worst, and it was always a false image of who I really was. So, I didn't actually get to go through school as myself. It was like an imposter. Wasn't me. And I always - always - had such a difficult time accepting it. I kept pushing for the real Leah, this is who I really am, this is who I'm going to be today. And I would try to project that person, and try to re-convince people over and over again "this is who I am—whatever it is you saw the other day, that's not me—this is who I am!" Sometimes I wake up okay, I'm reborn today. I remember switching schools several times like oh, yay, now I have an opportunity to be reborn again, now people can see who I really am. Now I can really live to my fullest potential and I won't be bogged down by these strange disorders that I deal with every day. It was debilitating, socially. I remember having crushes on guys, trying to talk to them, and the more I liked the guy the less we actually interacted, and the harder it was for me to spend any time out. I even remember one day I wanted to kind of set things straight, because weird rumors had gone around that I'm really in love with this guy, and we didn't even really know each other, so I remember pulling him aside. I had written out what it is that I wanted to say. I literally had to have a script in order to talk to him, because I knew that if I didn't have a script and I tried to do it by memory or I tried to do it on the spot, like improvise, not only would I not have much to say, but anything that would come out was gonna sound ridiculous, and I was going to look ridiculous because the way that I would communicate would be all messed up. I'm sure I would have stuttered, would have messed up my words, would have had these awkward pauses, so I literally wrote it out, and the first thing I had to do was explain that I didn't want to forget what it is I wanted to say, so that I wouldn't seem ridiculous that I have this, like, sheet of notes in order just to talk to the guy that I had a crush on.

Question: How old were you then?

Sixteen, fifteen. By then, wouldn't you think I'd have a little more self-control? No, I wasn't just a fumbling eleven-year-old having my first crush, no, I was almost an adult and still couldn't even carry a conversation with a guy that I didn't know very well.

Question: What would you say has been the hardest part of living with Lyme?

My inability to communicate effectively. Even though I have already told the whole story on how difficult it was for me to just have a normal conversation with somebody in the situation where I might be nervous, you have to think how often we use speech, how much talking we do in a life. Think about a school situation when you're in class you're asked to share your thoughts - you raise your hand, you make a comment, you ask a question, you have to get up, you have to do presentations in the social settings. You're talking with people, you're talking to people you don't know very well, you're talking with people that make you nervous. How can you live a normal life if you can't talk normally, if any time you are nervous in any way whatsoever, not even just nervous, excited, like even if I was gonna get together with my friends, who I was comfortable with. When I would first get together with them I was excited to see them, so I always remembered in the beginning I had this kind of impairment about my way of talking. I would kind of get stuck, or would take me a second to gather my thoughts, or when it would come out, it's kind of like my mouth jiggled a little bit, or my eyes always felt kind of weird, like my eyes would hurt. You wouldn't be a be able to see it necessarily, but I always felt like my eyes were moving, or like jiggling. The more nervous I was, the more of just my face, mouth, nerves, everywhere, behind my neck, my shoulders, the whole chest area, which is where your central nervous system is always, felt funny, fuzzy. You can't be normal. I did a good job putting on a show, and acting, pretending that I felt normal, but I seldom did. I had to be totally, totally relaxed in order to function mostly normally.

Question: So, you lived so many years with Lyme—when did you find out that that you still had it?

Let's see, it was pretty soon after I got married, and we had moved to Maryland. I believe it was 2009-2010. It was 2010. So that was four years ago, so I would have been 24. I believe it was in November, my first Lyme appointment was November, so I had just turned 25. I picked up Lyme when I was three. That's more than 20 years carrying the disease in my body. It's not just a rash and achy joints. That's what most people think Lyme disease is. Maybe when you first pick it up, the very first symptoms as it's going through your blood, if it's just your blood that's infected, that's how you might respond. But the longer it's in your body, the deeper it goes, and the more areas of your body it's going to infect, so that's the reason why the symptoms that I had as I was an older youth were different than the symptoms that I had when I was a young child. Treated for three weeks, yeah, cleaned my blood system out, that's why I felt better. That's why my achy joints went away. You always look good, fine, but it's all those other strange things that you carry that can be so easily misdiagnosed as other things. Those are the signs that there's something else still going on, and those are the harder things to detect. For a long time, most doctors didn't even consider it.

Question: So, how did you find out that you still had Lyme?

My dad.

My dad was the one that, in way, saved me. His mother saved him, and he saved me. He was treated for Lyme, and he had been undergoing intense treatment for quite a while, I believe a couple of years by the time he suggested that I get tested, because not only do my dad and I have very similar personalities, but the ways in which my dad struggled, they're all most of his life very similar to the ways in which I struggled. So, once he started to get better, and he was healthy enough to even be able to think to maybe see if anybody else he knows might be sick, he recognized similarities and urged me to get tested again, this time at IGeneX. So, I had my first appointment. It was this long consultation and I was asked about "do you have this," "do you experience this," "what about when this happens," and the more questions that were asked the more I'm like, these are all common occurrences for me, these are symptoms of Lyme.

Well, it already seems pretty apparent that I have a lot of the symptoms, and when I got tested, it came back positive for Lyme antibodies. Now *antibodies* is not the infection itself; now, I'm not a doctor, so I may not be seeing this to the most effective way, but the antibodies are expressing that Lyme was at least in my body at some point. And apparently the antibodies were high enough where it was considered a positive test result. And this wasn't just any old tests; I didn't just go to a regular old lab get my blood tested for Lyme, and that's why I know I got what is on my test. No, it had to be packaged up and shipped to California to IGeneX. And once it was tested at IGeneX, that's where the testing was sensitive enough to be able to check the antibodies. So, I remember, I had Lyme when I was four, at least I was treated when I was four, so antibodies after more than 20 years? You think maybe I still have it? Yeah. So, that's how I found out I still had Lyme.

And once you go so long thinking you don't have it, and you're told over and over again, well, you have this, and you have this, and this is what's wrong with you. I remember it took almost a year before it really sunk in that I still had it. Becomes part of your identity, you know, the disorders that you're told you have, and always feeling like though there's just something wrong with me.

Question: After re-discovering that you still had Lyme, how long did you get treated for?

Three years. A long time. And it took a year before I actually started to feel improvement. If anything, I felt worse at first. I started off with several symptoms from what I remember being kind of on a minor level, aside from the anxiety and the nausea and the speech impediment, but all the rest of the symptoms, anything that was just bodily discomfort, they were kind of small. But once I started the antibiotics, started to grow, got bigger, got worse, and I started even feeling symptoms that whether or not I had them at all to begin with, it was almost as if I didn't even know I had them. Maximized it. Made me feel more.

Question: Do you recall what kind of medicine you took?

Sure. I was treated with several, and I had to try different concoctions until I got the right one, but I started off with the classic amoxicillin, and nothing else for a little while. The first doctor that I had did not treat me aggressively, and then Rifampin was added, and once I started the Rifampin, that's when I started to feel different, that's when the symptoms started to increase. It's almost like I started to swell. And I was treated on that for a while, I believe I even started to feel a tiny bit of improvement. I don't remember what else was added, but I do remember that the first medicine that I took that really started to make me feel different was the Malarone, and that made me sicker. I think at that point in my treatment after about two years by then, it really hit my nerves. I had a lot of nausea, dizziness, and granted the antibiotics make you feel that way to begin with, but it felt as if it was pulling the infection to the surface. And then because it was, I was just too dizzy, so switched to Coartem, and the Coartem is what did it. Once I started the Coartem, I really started to feel a difference; an improvement. The way that I described it when I actually started to really heal, was my whole life, I felt like a television that wasn't coming in very well, that was fuzzy, fuzzy.... That's the way that I experienced my life, that's how I saw things through my eyes, that's how I experience things through my body, and how I would respond to life stress, to excitement.

Once I started to get better, it was as if I was living life in High Definition (HD). Everything just kind of cleared out. The fuzziness just subsided, and there was this incredible stillness. I was so used to the fuzziness, it was as if I was a child growing up that had never seen a clear television. Now I was seeing life in HD! I'm still getting used to it. Everybody loves this story: I was so used to being nervous and anxious and shaky, intense, nauseous, that when I actually have experiences that make me really upset or nervous, like going and having my blood taken, I'll be sitting there having my blood taken, and oh crap - here it comes - the wave of nausea, the adrenaline is gonna hit me any moment - and yeah, happens a little bit, but then, I'm just sitting there anticipating it, and anticipating, anticipating, and nothing happened. I kind of look to the right, I kind of look to the left, and I realized that oh, it's not gonna happen, and I just get up and I walk out. Whereas, years ago when I was getting my blood taken I would get hit with the wave of adrenaline.

Once it's actually happening because I've been so anxious up until that moment, and then afterwards it's kind of like I would try to get the adrenaline to just clear out, and I would have to either like sit back, or I'd sometimes sit with my head in between my knees, because somehow bringing the blood to my head would make the blood not rush into the part of my body that makes me nauseous. And it would take me sometimes 15 to 20 minutes to calm down. Sometimes I'd throw up, sometimes I didn't, so just to be able to go in and get my blood work and be able to just get right up and walk out was something I had never experienced. I was never afraid of the needle, I was afraid of the anxiety and nausea. It didn't bother me that it pricks for a second; really I'm not all that squeamish when it comes down to it, but my body would just overreact so much, I was just terrified of what my body was going to do and lose my lunch. I don't like to lose my lunch.

Question: What would be your advice to anybody that is going through Lyme, or anybody that knows somebody that's going through Lyme, what would you say would be the best way to to overcome it, or to at least start?

I would say first thing anybody should do, especially if you think you might have Lyme is to seriously consider that you might. Even if you have been tested, and it has come back negative, if you are experiencing multiple symptoms, you need to take it seriously and get tested at IGeneX, especially if you live in a heavily Lyme populated area. Now it's spreading to the point where it's everywhere, but if you're up north, New Hampshire, Connecticut, Massachusetts, Maine, Vermont, you better take it seriously. Become aware. First step is openness. Second step is awareness. Learn what it means to have Lyme disease. Learn what it means to have *chronic* Lyme disease, and the difference between when you are first infected and if you have been infected for a long, long time. Whether it's a couple of months or if it's been years that you've been feeling this, your symptoms though more extreme might differ from person to person. Each person's body responds differently. For me, aside from the very beginning, I had very little pain. This was not a painful disease for me. It was almost all neurological and psychological. Nerves. I always felt like a nervous wreck. That was the indicator. And it was irrational. I would really over-respond to things that shouldn't have made me that anxious and that sick. And for people that think they might have Lyme, or know somebody that has Lyme symptoms, which are many, just learn about it. Get tested. Go to a Lyme-literate doctor; not your typical infectious disease doctor. Go to a Lyme specific doctor or LLMD. Don't just get tested at a typical lab. If you go in and you have a consultation with a Lyme specialist, and you have several of the symptoms, you need to get tested at IGeneX because IGeneX is a lab that actually tests thoroughly, whereas average labs don't.

And then you need to stick to your protocol and a doctor that is willing to treat you as long as it takes to get *better*. And from what I've learned meeting other people with chronic Lyme disease - long-term Lyme disease - it usually requires many months or even years of treatment. Some people get treated for seven, eight, nine months, and then relapse. Well, sure. Because by that time it, started to get deeper into your body, you're going to feel improvement. But in order for it to get as deep as your bones—this is a stubborn infection—it takes a long time. Meet other people who have Lyme, who have had Lyme and been cured. And don't just go to a family practitioner and ask them about Lyme and take what they say about Lyme to be the truth. I think in almost any serious medical condition, it is not going to be known automatically how a disease really works. Look at cancer. Think about when doctors first started really learning about cancer, how it was treated. You could also consider and compare AIDS. It takes time to understand the disease, especially if it affects people differently. So, unless you are going and you're talking to somebody that is incredibly aware of Lyme disease and has done their work and studied it, and treated people and cured people, don't just take what you hear.

Question: Is there any final message you have for anyone watching this video about understanding Lyme?

I would say when it comes to learning about Lyme disease, I'm becoming aware of what it does and how it affects the body, how it affects your life. It's just one step that leads to the other steps to understanding a greater problem. Lyme disease is just one disease that people, professionals, are still trying to understand as so many people are still ignorant about it. There are so many more problems within the medical industry. We could list so many. For me, having Lyme disease has just confirmed that this world can be really screwed up. Things are not always as they seem. And sometimes man's needs, humanity's needs, are overlooked. I would suggest to anybody to just be open; that what you think you may know about Lyme disease, about other diseases, about the whole medical industry, how humans are cared for, may not be what you think."

***

EXCLUSIVE INTERVIEW: NH Land Surveyor, Henry H. Amsden

My father, Henry H. Amsden, a land surveyor in the states of New Hampshire and Maine since the mid 1970's, spent more time than most in the fair woods of New England for many decades. The family business established as H.H. Amsden & Sons Land Surveyors generated over 5,000 maps of property depicting boundary and subdivisions for individuals and businesses. During the early years, encounters with ticks as a result of these forays into the wilderness were infrequent but not unheard of. As the years advanced, there was a noted increase in tick population, and the exposure to this increased as well. Where the occasional tick encounter was uncommon in the early days, with increasing frequency we often found not one but several ticks pulled from our clothes or skin. While the spread of Lyme disease was quietly making its way into the northern woods of New England, we were vaguely aware of this but not alarmed as there was little reason for fear based upon what was known at the time.

Cases of Lyme were a rare occurrence, and it was even more rare to read of it in the paper or see something about it on the news. Neatly tucked out of view, we took it in stride, as an insignificant part of the daily battle with insects; black flies, deer flies, mosquitoes and hornet nests being more of a concern. My brothers and I were used to the heat, rain, cold, insects, poison ivy and dense undergrowth that accompanied our trips to the woods, and we thought little of it other than being a typical part of everyday life as a surveyor.

When my aunt was diagnosed with multiple sclerosis during the mid-1980's, the possibility it came from an infected tick was never considered by her doctors. When my daughter Leah was diagnosed with "juvenile arthritis" in the early 1990's, this too was never considered by her doctors as a possibility. Tick-born infections as a probable source of my general deterioration over the period during the 1970's to the 1990's also was never considered, and thousands of others just like us from all over New England were largely ignored and continue to be misdiagnosed. Why some people succumb to the disease and others don't is one of the many remaining mysteries of this disease, and from the enormous amount of anecdotal evidence there is a high probability that *many* people have it but are unaware of it.

It was nearly too late by the time I was accurately diagnosed, and by then I had lost everything, including the ability to work or make a living.

However my dad, Henry, appeared to continue in generally good health in spite of the high probability of having also contracted babesia. But suddenly in 2010 he succumbed to a severe and acute condition that landed him in the emergency room. With uncontrollable shakes and fever, he was quickly admitted to the ICU at the local hospital and setup with heavy IV doses of undisclosed antibiotics. When the attending physician learned that he had very recently experienced an encounter with a tick embedded in his forearm, he quietly diagnosed the episode first as *sepsis*, a diversionary term used to avoid revealing the truth behind tick-borne infections and suggested "*babesia*" as a possible diagnosis. Within 24-36 hours, the episode had passed.

But this was not the first episode. He had a similar episode some months earlier, where again, the typical response of the medical community was one of standard denial and feigned ignorance. A couple of months later, it took a third incident for physicians to finally face the reality, at significant cost to taxpayers, insurance, hospital care and patients alike, to say nothing of the misery and suffering endured.

In his own words, here is the account of Henry's written testimony:

May 5, 2015: At age 74 in 2010, physically active and in documented good health.

FIRST SCENARIO: EARLY-MID 2010

1. Bad deer tick surgically removed, mid-April (no test for Lyme done on tick or on me). Two doxycycline tablets given and taken. Record made of tick removal.

2. Mid-July (about 3 months later), extremely hot day. Met crew in the field and did a little minor digging. Sent crew home, per heat. In air conditioned circumstances otherwise during day. Ate spaghetti (?!) in back yard late evening, fell blah, not sick, just sub-blah. 9 P.M., after urinary relief returned to couch and, suddenly, with no warning whatsoever, went into what docs call "RIGOR," pronounced "RYE-GORE" not as in "REEGORE", as in rigorous activity. This was clearly a violent, epileptic-level of shaking chills. No number of piled on blankets sufficed. Points to remember: a) session lasted 20-30 minutes, b) shaking (which, of course, Mom observed) was violent enough to tear or stretch a muscle in my left shoulder. This was bad enough to have the Infectious Disease doc at the hospital observe me for spinal meningitis, which thankfully was not indicated [I told them I pulled my shoulder!]. c) We decided to tough out the night, which passed un-eventfully. However, next morning, the entire bed was drenched, pillow, sheets, blanket, etc., with more water than I would have believed could issue from one-middle-sized human being. I don't remember being thirsty.

3. Urine had wispy clouds of whitish-swirls observable.

4. Visited family physician mid-day, urine tested bad for bacteria, started on more doxycycline, blood taken but no results available then, and told to go to ER if chills returned.

5. Circa.11-12 P.M. that night, rigor returned and, again (I think this is of seminal importance) lasted the same 20-30 minutes.

6. In ER, got first shot of some 'industrial strength' anti-biotics and started feeling fine but kept for 3 nights. Probably started saline

IV water drip; that's pretty standard now-a-days.

7. Tests showed infection had settled into kidneys, with apparent severe level of sepsis (?).

8. Next 3 nights uneventful, except couldn't sleep to the point of beginning to hallucinate on the last night (that was most unpleasant).

9. On oral-antibiotics for the next few weeks and returned immediately to normal activity.

SECOND SCENARIO: OCTOBER, 2010

1. After evening drive, with no prior symptoms, returned at dusk and had abnormal joint pain, like arthritis.

2. Again, late evening, don't remember whether in bed or not, sudden return of extreme rigor.

3. Lasted 20-30 minutes. (Mom wanted to take me to the ER before they stopped, but the thought of moving or even the slightest skin exposure was terrifying.)

4. At ER, more higher-level 'industrial strength' anti-biotics and 2-3 more days in hospital.

5. This time, kidneys okay, but exhaustive x-rays showed lung shadow in back of heart. I remember, a week or so later, coughing some faint blood stains which did not appear again.

6. More oral anti-biotics after return to normal activity. NOTE: Since we went immediately to the ER, we don't know whether the same sweats would have returned if 'toughing' it out again 'til the next day.

THIRD SCENARIO: JUNE, 2011

1. Red spot appeared on inner side of upper right arm.

2. Dr. D. (both M.D. and "Naturpathic") could not see entry point but spot began to enlarge.

3. Will send the pix daily taken as the spot enlarged.

4. Put on out-patient anti-biotic IV for several days.

5. Spot gradually disappeared.

6. All normal activity since then.

MY HOPE FOR THOSE WHO READ THE ABOVE AND THE ACCOMPANYING INFO:

1. Local hospital gave absolutely no diagnosis on just what caused these 3 episodes, except, "yeah, you're some sick" (second scenario physician, a Bulgarian, good guy, said that when he saw the daily chart, I was the first dude he wanted to see that day).

2. Dr. D. wrote courteous letter to Dr. N.e (infectious disease specialist, not a Lyme "believer") giving his best shot as BABESIOSIS.

3. D. also supervised complete, exhaustive application to Igenix lab, which came back negative, except one or two minor titers which he discounted. This, of course, was after I had been pumped full, via 2 sessions, of all kinds, varieties and levels of super anti-biotics. Does this affect a subsequent Lyme test? Dunno.

4. I retrieved about every scrap of paper from everybody which I have in a fat binder.

5. Don't know why anyone who is curious should not have access to same. I'm getting too old to be fussy about such things. Can scan all and forward.

6. WANT VERY MUCH TO KNOW IF ANYONE HAS HAD SIMILAR EXPERIENCES, LYME DISEASE, BABESIOSIS OR NOT.

7. If someone has had similar experience, hopefully they'll share same with me, privately/anonymously if they wish.

EVERYONE, ESPECIALLY THE MEDICAL COMMUNITY AND THE LYME PEOPLE NEED TO KNOW IF THE ABOVE EXPERIENCES ARE CONSISTENT WITH ANY KNOWN HUMAN ILLNESS.

***

Following is the actual transcripts of interview testimony recorded by Victor Fontane, Leah's husband, in 2015, and published on *The Lymester* YouTube Channel:

Exclusive Interview with NH Land Surveyor Henry Amsden (Transcript)

"A Tick Encounter with Babesia"

From YouTube Channel:

The Lymester

Published on May 23, 2015

Question: What is your first and last name?

"My first name is Henry, my last name is Amsden.

Question: Where were you born and raised?

I was born in Concord New Hampshire in a hospital, but I was raised in the town of Hill, New Hampshire.

Question: Do you have any children?

We have three sons, yes.

Question: Are you married?

Very much so. (Laughs.)

Question: You have Lyme, or did you have Lyme in the past?

You've asked the right question. The only diagnosis that I have was from a naturopathic MD; he's also not just a naturopathic, but he's also full MD and that was *babesiosis,* which is one of the co-infections of the Lyme filled tick, as we say.

Question: When did you find out you had this infection?

I found out something was terribly wrong, which would have been in July of 2010.

Question: Do you still have the infection?

No one knows. All I can tell you is this, there is a history to how this came about which is quite simple if you want to have it related here. I'm a land surveyor. I have to work out into the woods of New Hampshire where there are known many, many ticks. Every other tick in New Hampshire and southeastern New Hampshire has Lyme disease in it, and I was bitten by a tick in April of 2010. Fortunately for the record, I couldn't get all of the mouth or parts of the tick out and I had it surgically removed, which gives a paper trail. And so it was surgically removed at my doctor's office and I was of course given a record of this and the woman who took it out says, oh yes, this is one of the bad ones.

She handed me, very daintily, what remained of it. I didn't want to get anywhere near it. Er, ah, after that experience when I was there they gave me two pills, that's it. And then what happened later, I'm sure you'll get to that but at least I had proof that I had been bitten by a tick, however, the tick was not analyzed, so did it have Lyme? I don't know. I might add to this that most people assume that if you are treated within 24 hours of a tick bite, then you won't get Lyme disease. I think it may have been possibly less than 24 hours when they gave me the two pills, well so, like the next day or so, so the exact number of hours I already can't tell you, but it could be as much as 24 hours.

Question: Anybody else know about this infection?

All we knew this time is simply that I'd been bitten by a tick. I did not have the bullseye rash, nothing until next July gave me any reason to think that I had anything at all. I was just as normal as ever.

Question: If you could explain to me while you're going through this situation, how did you feel about it?

The only way I can answer is to explain what happened in July. I can't precisely date, but about July 15, 2010, very hot day in New Hampshire, so hot that I sent my crew home that were working for me. I was an in air-conditioned car, went into an air-conditioned office, did go out in the heat a little bit, but nothing unusual, nothing strenuous. Everything was fine until that evening. The only thing I remember, about six o'clock, I felt malaise, not serious except just blah, which is not unusual; thought nothing of it. Ate supper at nine o'clock, got up to go to the bathroom, just the usual call, came back, and then it began – bang! I have to tell you what happened because I'm hoping it may help someone else, and the magic word as far as I know is *babesiosis.* There are several co-infections from Lyme disease, and two or three others that I can't pronounce, but this one of them is babesiosis. It is a Paramecium type, not a virus, but it's very similar to malaria, and it's in there, you can get it. At any rate, nine o'clock came, and then what happened to me was almost like an epileptic fit of chills. No, not frothing at the mouth or thrashing on the floor, but a sense that I was cold and absolutely uncontrollable. I was thrashing around and got into bed, my wife put covers on me and still I felt cold. And there I found that the medics have a word for this, it's called *rigor*, same spelling, but it's a medical term for extreme chills. These were very extreme; it just completely took over. It was like a thunderbolt. This is not like chronic Lyme disease, but all of a sudden you're fine and the next minute feels you are dying. The interesting thing, this lasted approximately just a half an hour, so this brought us up to close to ten o'clock. Well, we didn't know what to do. I hoped it wouldn't come back.

We decided to tough it out for the evening. I noted that my urine that night looked like 'mushroom soup.' Whatever happened got to my kidneys, as the next morning I got up and I would not believe that a human being could get rid of such moisture by sweating - everything was soaked. I don't mean wet, damp, but soaked, I mean really soaked. I must have been dehydrated, so I went to the doctor. Having a fever of about 101 degrees, so of course they started me on a regimen of doxycycline, which is for Lyme. They started me on that and they said if it happens again, go to the ER. Home we went. About midnight, the same violent shaking, almost epileptic chills, no control over my motions. It was so violent that I pulled a muscle, wrenched and/or tore it, and when I got to the hospital, the infectious disease doctor came in to check me for meningitis, I told him no. I told him it's nothing to do with that. Now this is odd - they started shooting antibiotics into me, and far as I'm concerned, I was ready to go home. I was in the hospital three days, no more shaking, so after this three days went home. Was fine until October, of course that's several months later. Felt fine and been busy doing my work, no problems at all, until in the middle of October we took a ride just to get out, and suddenly had very unusual arthritic type pain, almost about the same time, around nine o'clock, bang! The same rigor, violent, shaking chills and shaking to the point almost like an epileptic does. This time we didn't wait; right up to the emergency room. Interestingly enough, they started me on antibiotics probably about midnight. The next day when my doctor came in that morning he looked at the chart and he says 'oh, that's the guy I'm going to look at first,' something about the symptoms concerned them, so of course they started me on antibiotics. I had shaking chills, nothing, however on the X-ray, they thought it had gotten into the lungs this time. This is what's weird, whatever it is weakening the system so that the term they use 'opportunistic bugs' can come in and move in, so if it's the Lyme babesiosis that's doing it, all it's doing is weakening my system so something else that's hanging around can jump in and take over.

This time he took a lot of x-rays and thought there was a slight shadow in back of the lung. Kidneys were fine, everything else is fine, so they assume that this time had gone into the lungs. A few days later at the hospital I did cough up very faint bit of blood, so this is consistent with pneumonia, or what they thought was pneumonia, so this time they used 'industrial-strength' antibiotics. Three days later I'm out of the hospital, and the only thing left in the story is my naturopathic doctor, whom I saw shortly thereafter. There was no diagnosis for this. Nobody said, 'well, why did this happen?' So how do i know it's not going to happen again? What's wrong with me? 'Oh, we fixed you.' That's all. This is very tacky; they have to be careful what they say. They all knew ahead of course I had a tick removed back in April, so you know it's not up to them to say 'well then, you've got Lyme disease,' but I was obviously concerned because we have Lyme disease in the family.

I found this naturopathic doctor right in Concord, fully-fledged MD, but also naturopathic but specializing in Lyme, and sent my blood sample to IGeneX in Palo Alto, California. That lab has the most sophisticated tests for Lyme or chronic Lyme, came back negative. So, what happened to the Lyme disease? Well, not long after being pumped full of industrial-strength antibiotics, I wouldn't think it would show anything. At any rate, there was no more tests. He looked it over very carefully and gave me a nice letter which he sent to the infectious disease doctor at Concord Hospital. He sent a nice two-page letter, 'my best diagnosis is babesiosis.' That is all we have. One thing I'd like to throw in here, I read in Pamela Weintraub's book, it's kind of a Bible for Lyme disease—something about a group of surveyors on Cape Cod. This would probably in the 70s, and they all came down with babesiosis, no, not Lyme disease, not the co-infections or all those other strange things, but babesiosis, an easy name to remember. I have yet been able to find out what happened to these guys, what was it like, what were their symptoms and all that stuff, so here I am all alone with this one little diagnosis, babesiosis.

Do I know that I have Lyme disease? No, I do not. All I know is what I told you here. Nothing has happened since.

Question: Did anyone else know of your ordeal, other than your wife, what you were going through?

I don't think there's anybody I didn't let know, especially where we had Lyme disease in the family. However, my understanding of the other three members of my family was genuine Lyme disease, the long 'chronic' variety. There's nothing chronic about this, this was acute to the nth power, you know, *bang*! Like earlier in July, *bang* in October. Well, that's not Lyme disease. When people get 'regular' Lyme, sometimes, but apparently not often, there's a bull's-eye rash, they have aches and pains and a rather gradual deterioration usually over weeks, usually not something acute like this, and that's about all I can tell you.

Question: So, what was the reaction of those who knew what you had and what you were going through?

"Gee, we're sorry for you." This is perhaps one of the reasons I'm glad you're doing this. I have on the net tried to read the symptoms of babesiosis, and yes, serious, violent, shaking chills and a few other things that correspond to what I had, but I still would like to interface with some people who have had the same experiences, or similar, where they were certain or had some diagnosis right off the bat that was the babesiosis. They took my blood of course over at the hospital, but they didn't send it to Palo Alto, California (IGeneX Lab), they don't do that at the hospitals, only my naturopathic doctor did this, and this was after the second episode where I'd been thoroughly zapped with high speed antibiotics.

Question: Did you know about Lyme and babesiosis before all this happened?

I hardly knew the word babesiosis, but we've known about the Lyme ever since my second granddaughter was diagnosed with Lyme disease in approximately nineteen ninety when she was four years old, so we've known about Lyme disease and been conscious of that at least from then on. And then of course my oldest son, and then my youngest son, both diagnosed with chronic Lyme disease and treated accordingly.

Question: Has this experience changed you in some way, physically or otherwise?

Scared of the cold! Really, I think this is probably just psychological, but when I get cold, start to tremble a little bit, I'm always afraid that's gonna come back again. Well, it's improbable, so that's psychological, and I'm of such an age where some of the aches and pains are normal, I mean after all, we're land surveyors. If there was something more, maybe I could be more helpful. That's all.

Oh, I think I mentioned that no one ever told me what was wrong with me in the hospital, no one said well, maybe you've got Lyme, and of course we have to mention the huge controversy over this, country-wide and beyond our country, that is whether there is such a thing as chronic Lyme disease. Well, if I had Lyme disease, most certainly was not chronic, so I'm not really in that cycle, but my two sons and granddaughter are in that chronic Lyme. Whether it's 'chronic Lyme,' whether there is such a thing or not, I can tell you this much - my second granddaughter, her experience is worth retelling if this is the place to do it. I don't have to name her (see Leah Fontane's testimony in her interview) necessarily, she was about four. Shortly before this time they were in Enfield, Connecticut, and camped out on a lawn there, had a good time and all that, and of course is not very far from Lyme, Connecticut, so this would probably be in 1989 or so.

Not long after, her health began to deteriorate where she could not walk and they had to pick her up and carry her. Well, for a four-year-old child, this doesn't happen unless there is something wrong - you can't stop them from walking.

So, they went to a doctor. I have the records, the general records, this would have been about January of 1990 - I believe all kinds of earth anti-arthritic drugs were tried, or some psychotropic. In other words, you know, "it's all in her head," she's jealous of big sister, or that kind of thing. This is a typical syndrome that when doctors don't understand something, sometimes they think that the kid is faking it or something. There's a classic example of this which I'll just throw in here of a guy who did have Lyme who went through about 20 doctors or so, I'm exaggerating perhaps some, but they finally sent him to a psychiatrist. The psychiatrist took one look at him and said "What are you doing here? You're sick!" This is what we're getting at. So, this went on for several months with virtually no improvement into late nineteen ninety.

Somewhere along probably July or so, when the child's father asked his doctor who had been treating her since the beginning of 1990 about having a Lyme test, and then didn't think about it. For reasons that had nothing to do with my granddaughter or them, they happen to have changed doctors - I think he was orthopedic, and they handed the case over to a family physician. And so a couple of months later, after the Lyme test was had been ordered by the child's father, they met with the new physician. He opened up the folder and said, 'Oh, what are you doing for the Lyme disease?" It had come back positive and they were never notified! Oh yes, we remember this the time, I remember going and visiting her when her mother went in with her and so forth; she was in the hospital. She was put into the hospital, given IV antibiotics, and according to the report the recovery was not instantaneous, but a matter of days and she seemed to be as good as new. But there's a catch. There's a saying amongst Lyme people, and this based on a great deal of evidence, once those bugs are in, if you do not zap them immediately, they get in, and they stay in. They go into the flesh, the organs, the muscles, the sinews and so forth, and it's quite possible you may never get them out. But if you're not aware whether you have been treated properly and sufficiently, there needs to be a follow-up antibiotic treatment if you're going to really get them all. This was not done in the case of my second granddaughter, and over the next 20 years, oh yes, there are a great number of symptoms that were not discovered until only a couple years ago when she had the IGeneX test which came back positive. But if you let it go, you're already a little late.

Question: What happened to your oldest son?

My oldest son may have lost the following to Lyme disease: an excellent job, all his real estate, his marriage, and his health. We noticed it probably close to ten years ago while they were living in Hopkinton near Concord, had their own house, doing very well, both of them, had good jobs, he had an excellent job in with a school system where he was the one who connected and made sure the computers all talk to each other, wonderful future. Two things: he complained that his feet were cold, all the time and that 'nothing seemed to work,' and he kept saying "I'm gonna be out of a job, I'm just going to be out of a job." No, but he wouldn't say why, what's wrong. It was a nice job. To jump ahead a little bit, I got a phone call some number of months after this and says 'hi dad, how you doing?'

I replied "Well, what are YOU doing?"

"I'm sitting on a tractor in Florida."

A lot of the strange things that happened seemed to me to result for what turned out to be a positive chronic Lyme result from IGeneX, but this was only after going through many doctors, many medicines, and until that came back and he got with a good Lyme doctor now here in Florida, there was very grave concern what was going to happen.

Question: And your younger son?

There's one parallel here. He walked out of an excellent job, and it was obvious something was wrong. Then lost his house, which did not need to happen. And one of the key things I knew something was wrong is when he had certain friends, one of his neighbor as it were, used to help him. Just a good guy. And he started shedding friends also, and that was not, that was not good. We had a naturopathic person who finally persevered and sent his blood into IGeneX, and I believe she told him that the result was raging stage 2 chronic Lyme disease. That's not all, he went back and had the regular CDC test approved by FDA and that was positive also. The results were a mixed bag. He did not respond to antibiotics as good as my oldest son, but the damage persisted. Another simple example: in the midst of all this, right, he lost his job, needed money crazily to just keep the houses. You got him a job at a local factory, good money, at least to start with, well, he couldn't handle it. The noise, confusion, and so forth, the psychological effect of whatever the bug does to you affected his ability to work in a noisy or confusing environment, even when he needs the money desperately. That's a general outline of my youngest son.

Question: So, what is his status now? Has he had, or currently in, additional treatment?

The Lyme treatment has been on and off, sometimes he's gone to the same naturopathic doctor that I spoke of earlier, and my understanding is that the good Lyme doctors are very attentive to your symptoms. Well, so much what the blood says, and this and that, but what do these people tell them, and this doctor took him off antibiotics, but he's going to have him test it again by IGeneX. Again, anyone who is familiar with Lyme knows these are *murky waters* even for the best Lyme doctors, and for most of the obviously symptomatic patients it *still* is murky waters, and people are beginning to recognize that. The other side of the coin, the CDC is slowly beginning to recognize there is such a thing as 'chronic Lyme disease.' Of course a number of us who have had it know that, but they're slowly starting to recognize it as well. I probably should mention in New Hampshire, I helped the effort. My whole family helped to get a law through which is on the books now, that you cannot prosecute a doctor for malpractice because he's giving more than the 30 days antibiotic. You can't go after him simply because he's going beyond the guidelines of 30 days from the given CDC guidelines.

If they have made their diagnosis that they believe it is Lyme disease, the doctor believes that then they are entitled to go beyond the

CDC guidelines and give antibiotics beyond their guidelines. That's at the moment the end of it; that's where it stands.

We have a lot of deer and moose in New Hampshire. My wife found this in print: sometimes they'll have a hundred thousand ticks on them when they are killed, or before they're killed. And to carry this one step further, there is an island off of Maine where a lot of deer on the island are having all kinds of troubles with ticks and Lyme disease and so forth, so they decided to kill all the deer. No more ticks, no more Lyme disease. The lesson is so obvious, that the large animals such as a deer or moose are acting as a vehicle, while the ticks' chances are much greater they're going to bite a white-footed mouse, and get the Lyme disease. The tick supposedly is born sterile, don't have Lyme disease or anything, and it lives as three feedings, three seasons. If it doesn't get to a white-footed Mouse in those three season, there's no Lyme, but with zillions of ticks, more and more of them are apt to get to the white-footed Mouse. And now we're being told that every other tick in southern New Hampshire has the Lyme bacteria in it. There's an unpleasant, obvious point here: these large animals are supporting, enabling, the ticks to multiply. This is a big problem. We have a Fish and Game Department to keep the deer and fish population thriving so people will come in and buy hunting and fishing licenses, buy gas and stay in motels and buy supplies and support our economy. It's not really because we love deer and love fish, well, some of us do just because they are fish and deer, but there is the economic basis for the management of Wildlife, and this is just a brutal truth of modern society.

Question: So, in your opinion, what do you think is the hardest part for people that contract these infections? I know that having the disease itself is very hard on the body and the mind, what about how it affects their life, how it affects other people in their life, where it takes them, if it's not treated?

I'm going to answer it this way - imagine that you're a healthy person. You're going along every day and all of a sudden you start bleeding someplace very, very slowly, and not enough so you think is anything seriously wrong. But you're bleeding a little bit faster than the blood is being replaced, so that it takes weeks maybe months before pretty soon you're getting so low on blood that you're in big trouble. That is a way to say the same thing about Lyme; that once it gets in it, starts sapping all the functions. This can just strictly seem to be only psychological, but the Lyme bugs can get into the brain as well. That's obviously very serious business. It can get into the heart muscles. The point is that this is nothing to be fooled with, this is a very serious thing because of its stealth. I think it's a good word. It is kind of a stealth disease. You can get bitten by the bug and doesn't happen like what happened to me, but you're starting to go downhill, and you've gone *a long way down hill before you know it*. This is what is so serious. And at that point it is *very difficult* to eradicate.

Question: Really interesting how a lot of the symptoms are very similar from person to person, but also how people can be affected very differently from the same problem.

I'm not a doctor, but after all, people are different, and they react differently. Some people are very sensitive, for example. Some people might be far more apt to react more violently to the Lyme bacteria than others, and that's just a difference in people. The Lyme itself and the bacteriological nature of it, there's a lot to learn yet. Well, you asked what can be done, number one, prevention, of course. Now, I'm under Medicare, and when I went in to the hospital those two times must have cost thousands of dollars. I never paid a nickel. The Lyme doctor sent this to IGeneX, eight hundred some odd dollars. I never paid a nickel. But that's not the story we're hearing of other people who have been bankrupted. For some people this has been a lifelong total disaster.

Here is an example:

A disabled child, her mother brought her in a wheelchair, she looked catatonic, eyes rolling. It is my understanding that the origin was Lyme disease. However, that child was given treatment three to four years ago, and she's now gained use of her legs. Before she was brought into the hearing in a wheelchair, but now she's an international swimming champion. For people who can't use their legs, whatever they did to help her had dramatic effect, because that poor child looked like she was not going to live very long. When we saw her on videotape, that I have at home and I'm sure it's around. There are a lot of strange stories out there, wonderful success stories, but for every success story there's some two or three or more of devastating destruction of people's lives.

Question: Why do you think it is so difficult when it comes to being able to get the resources, the antibiotics?

They are sometimes prohibitively expensive, so either way, it's a tough road if you do or think you have Lyme disease. This is something that I hope the people watching this will think about - the evidence for people being misdiagnosed for Lyme shows that they spent all kinds of money going from doctor to doctor, and different kinds of medications and so forth, over a long period of time before they finally found out it was Lyme. We're not treating them properly. Wait a minute! That cost a lot of money! Of course it did. Never mind the human agony. If you were able to diagnose it and treat it first, then you wouldn't be spending all that money that the insurance companies are forced to shell out. So, isn't there a simple solution that if Lyme is promptly treated and diagnosed and so forth, that you're doing away with some *huge* medical expenses that are going on as we speak. You can see my logic of this. It may be cheaper in the long run for the CDC to recognize it, and deal with it. Of course, you do understand the reluctance to prescribe antibiotics, because they're very concerned that antibiotics will become ineffective and new bugs will develop that are resistant to them. That may be so, but you can't tell that to someone who's dying of Lyme disease. They are the ones who need it, just like any kind of medicine that works; that has to be number one. How you control the overuse of antibiotics, I don't know, but helping to cure someone, or holding them in a good lifestyle who has Lyme is not overuse of antibiotics, in my view.

But somehow there has to be a simple way of saying look, we've got us a problem here, let's deal with it and not make these people go through endless agony before they find the right Lyme doctor. And then of course there is no reason why so many of the average doctors can't be doing this as well, without fear of retribution. But then of course the insurance companies, if they will support the purchase of antibiotics and so forth, then these people will be treated, and they won't have this huge expense that the insurance companies are already paying. Well, that's my point.

I should mention one other thing in this respect. This is really important. There are Lyme support groups anywhere and everywhere; you can go on the net and find them. There are some wonderful people who tell you where there is one. The minute you go in there, you're meeting other people like yourself, and you have a sense that you're not alone, and sooner or later you may find where to get the proper treatment, or where you can get the antibiotic that has been prescribed cheaper; that kind of thing. Sharing good information based upon experience. I've been to a couple of these with my oldest son, absolutely great, because it's very informal, and all of a sudden you've got other people like yourself that don't think you're crazy.

Question: What would be the best advice that you can give somebody that just found out that they have Lyme?

The chronic Lyme tick bite, the rash, the bullseye rash, this is my understanding - you can have terrible Lyme disease, sick as a dog, yet your tests are negative. And, you're going to have a few tests that's off the charts and you don't know it. Now, that may be the exception, but you have to be ready for this - I believe this can be documented.

Now your question again, as to the best advice that you can give these people to help them out of the situation, certainly go to your regular doctor. Get started, and if your family physician simply won't listen, at least you've got a paper trail started, you've got at least something. But go to a Lyme support group if you can find one, and find out where there is a Lyme doctor, even if you have to travel. And when it's not going to work with your local doctor, at least try the Lyme doctor rather than go to this whole long list of everything through psychotropic drugs, etc. before you try a Lyme doctor. So, in other words, there's no reason to wait to go through that. If you don't have Lyme, hopefully that Lyme doctor will be able to tell you – it may be something else, there are other diseases in the world other than Lyme disease. Well, this is a personal thing, but as you see God, get in touch with him, you can't go wrong. You may not have Lyme disease and you may not be cured of it, but I think it's wise to think, at least this is my view, the Creator permits these things, that doesn't mean that it's okay to endure them.

Beyond that, the simple things. First of all, prevention. Know what a tick looks like, know where they are be found, it's pretty well known now when you go out in the woods there are ways of tucking your boots in, there are anti-tick sprays, a whole panoply of things for prevention which I don't need to reiterate because it's well-known. You don't always know if you were bitten by a tick. Sometimes they will do their thing and drop off before you find out. But if the tick is on there, go to a doctor. And if you have the option of having that tick analyzed, do it. But, if you've been bitten, any of the regular doctors will give you the short-term antibiotic, and you may be clean as a whistle. Beyond that, you've got to be tuned into what are the chronic or long-term symptoms, or *anything* that seems out of whack in your life, like violent shaking chills as in my case. Then you know something's wrong with you, whether it's a tick that did it, hey, you're sick, do something about it. So, just general health you cannot go wrong. With general health, good exercise, diet, happiness - and that gets around to God again, but I won't go there."

***

PART 4

Cured from Advanced Late-Stage Chronic Lyme Disease

The following transcript is an inside view of having overcome the devastating personal struggle with advanced late-stage chronic Lyme disease. This insight reveals the "stealth" nature of Borrelia infection, some of the effects of neuro-borreliosis, and some incorrect myths about Lyme on the way to recovery. This interview is conducted by Victor Fontane of Eternal Lifetime Productions, LLC:

Cured from Advanced Late-stage Chronic Lyme Disease

(Transcript)

"The Lie Too Big To Admit"

From YouTube Channel:

The Lymester

Published on June 6, 2015

Stephen Amsden:

"I feel good. Probably the best of my adult life? And I'm fifty-five. It's been a long time. But, I've been thirteen months now pharm free—and that's p-h-a-r-m free; that's no antibiotics, no supplements, and I feel good. There's a clarity of mind that is there; the ability to focus. I can channel my energy, I have more energy, and the only drawback now is that I'm terribly out of shape from seven years of laying around on the couch, unable to do anything... but that's a small price to pay for having the clarity and focus of mind that has been missing for sooooo long, and it's nothing short of miraculous. And, it is living proof that you can recover, you can get your life back, you can be cured. Now, what is a cure? If you are 90% back, are you cured? Um… it remains to be seen. If it comes back next year or next month, well, are you still cured? Well, if you have the presence of mind… if you get 90% of your life back, you're having a quality of life way beyond your wildest imagination when you are sick, that goes a long ways to saying your cured. So, will I always be? I don't know, it's too early to tell, but for right now, has it been worth the 44 months of antibiotic treatment and the hell that you go through, hell ya! It's been thirteen months—that alone, just these 13 months have been worth it. So, anything here on out is gravy; it's gonna happen. And, here we go! I'm back! I'M BACK! And I'm doing stuff. Good stuff. And, it's with a new perspective; a perspective I wouldn't have had otherwise. Absolutely. And, would I go back and change anything? No. Just for the same reasons, here we are, these last 13 months, and this new perspective, is everything. So, life is good. Here we go!

Well, for the first time, I am who I am supposed to be, or who I really am. There are terrible identity issues for people with neuro-borreliosis, at least some of us, and the slow deterioration of your identify until you are no longer who you used to be at all, been stripped of all things that make up your personality; your ability to think—your faculties of will and reason—when those things are gone, there isn't much left. And I remember screaming at my doctor " I don't even know if I'm human anymore!" And that's what it felt like; I wasn't. It's not being human. The qualities that makes us humans are what make Lyme so diabolical, and to have those things back, I can rest now comfortably knowing that I am who I am, and that was not there for years, years, maybe even decades. So, on one hand you could look back and say, "I've lost my whole life to this," but on the other hand, you could say "I made it through the Swamp and I have my life back, I have *new* life, and a new opportunity to move on. So, who's to say, who's to say that anything could have been better? I suppose, sure, if I had never had it, I'd have had all those years to be who I am and maybe further ahead, but at the same time, who can say? You can't say that. Well, before, during the slow, gradual onset of the affliction there was a growing sense of being self-conscious *all the time*; nothing seemed right. I did not feel part of humanity. I felt separate, *separated* from it.

I often use the analogy of being stuck inside a "glass terrarium"; I could barely see through the glass to the outside world. That was my life for *years*, unbeknownst to me, for the longest period. Only in the past few years did I learn why and that this is *not* a natural thing. So, the difference is night and day; it couldn't be more antithetical now to what I was then.... really a mere apparition of a human before; I still say now that I was not human. I did not possess the characteristics of it; I did not have the feelings of empathy; and the reason and the will; none of the clarity; all that was gone, didn't exist. It's a surreal world, it's a true "reality"—not a pleasant one, it's a horrific one. I knew it at the time, but did not know that I would ever get out of it. This is where a lot of people fall short when on the long-term antibiotic treatment. They see that they are not getting well, they feel worse, and these are the things you need to keep in mind when you get on this path because, it's going to be a *long* time before you start feeling better. And you're going to feel a lot worse getting there. This is *normal*. This is normal for people who are severely compromised. This is what to expect. And still today, I see that people still do not understand that *duration* of treatment is as important as finding out what you've got, getting on the right protocol. If you don't have that duration of treatment, you *will* relapse, and you will fall back into.... (laughs) you will fall back! Into! (laughs again.)

The duration of the treatment is as critical as finding out. If you find out, get the right doctor, you get diagnosed properly, you get on the antibiotic protocol, but if you don't stay on that protocol long enough, it is all for naught. You might improve, you might get better, but if you do not stay with it 'til the bitter end... you have to stay on until you start feeling better. For me, that was forty-four months. Well, I've had it a long time. For some people it will take less; for some it will take more. Theoretically, every cell in the human body is replaced at my age every seven years, so the longest it could possibly take would be seven years to be completely free of this disease as long as you stay with it. The duration of treatment and the consistency... there are no "vacations" for people on antibiotics; you take two months off (for instance) your body is going to regenerate new cells that become re-infected, and basically you're starting over. And that may still be the case for me. If it's down in my bones and it comes back in two or three years, I may go back onto an antibiotic protocol to fight it, and I may never get rid of it. But, if I can maintain that 90% quality of life, then even with repeated treatment,

I still have a life worth living.

Number one, you find the right doctor. Number two, you get properly diagnosed. Number three, you get on the right antibiotic protocol, and number four, the duration of treatment—those are the four pillars of getting well. After that, it is maintenance. But, I would say the "fifth" pillar would be plain dumb luck. Most people are not as lucky as I am. I happen to have a support network through family who understood and was lucky enough to find a doctor who recognized the symptoms and got me on the path; and that the doctors I've had since being properly diagnosed, there have been two, were willing to take me the whole way home. They're not encouraging me to wrap up the 'ol antibiotics and start feeling better; they understood that the duration of treatment was equally as important as the other steps. So, I was extremely fortunate, and I may be only one out of a hundred people who will actually find out what they've got, find the right doctor, get the right protocol, and stay on it long enough to make the difference. I just don't see where there is much hope for the majority of people who are afflicted at this time, until we have a lot more knowledge and awareness out there. Most people will never find out what they've got; they'll be misdiagnosed with MS, Lupus, Parkinson's, Alzheimer's, any of the neuro-degenerative diseases that is probably the result of Lyme, and they call Lyme the Great Imitator, but I would call it the Great Initiator, for it is the source of many of these ailments.

The reason we're not seeing more progress on this is the *money*. It's all about the money. The health-care system is all about keeping people sick; healthy people don't pay, and diseased people do. There is no incentive in our medical health-care system to promote awareness about the cure for Lyme. They'll fight it tooth and nail because they've said it doesn't exist, they're making money on the fact that they don't have to disclose this information, and for them to come around and admit now that "oh, we were wrong," it's just not going to happen. Or. if it's going to happen, it's going to happen slowly. *The wheels of change turn slowly*, and that's what we're seeing here. It's a battle. It's a war. It's a global threat. There are probably a majority of the population that have it and *do not know it*. So, we have a long way to go; we've come a long way, but there's much further to go.

When we find out twenty years from now the truth about what's happening, phew, wow....and how many generations will have been born with it by then? It's incredible. Yeah, I mean, if we ignore the problem, it will become an extinction event. People will be so impaired being born with the disease, how will they even reproduce? And if they do, what kind of offspring after two or three generations; it's just not going to happen. So, the need for the awareness is critical, the need for treatment is critical, and we've got to stop fooling around and get together on this issue. There's no reason to deny people treatment when we know what works. And people who are battling that, I don't understand their motives other than self-interest and greed, and those are what are standing in the way.

There is such a thing as *normal*. People have often said that, "well, there's no such thing as normal" or normal is "relative," but there *is* a real normal. It's when your body is functioning the way that it should; that you're in good health; that autonomously you are functioning properly. Those things are normal. These are the things that people in the "normal" world take for granted. That you're able to multi-task, that you can *think* about things while you're *doing* other things; those things aren't happening for people with Lyme. Just to be normal again in this sense is the "Promised Land." It's heaven for us who have been through the hell. So, I would say that there is such a thing as Normal with a capital N, and it is where we want to be; that's where we *should* be; it's where we *need* to be, so that's what I am looking forward to is having a *normal* life—finally."

Proof Positive for Lyme: How I Was Cured

The YouTube Channel:

The Lymester

Published on June 8, 2015

Stephen Amsden:

"A person afflicted with Lyme is unlikely to get the help they need on their own. The gradual onset of the disease can impair judgment, reason, and the will, rendering the afflicted unable to act effectively on their own behalf. As the first and most important of the four steps to a cure is to find a Lyme-literate doctor, or LLMD, this is often done by a concerned family member or close friend. After nine or more misdiagnoses over thirty-three years, and testing for Lyme for the third time before finding the right doctor with the right diagnosis, it took another person to intervene on my behalf to make this happen. As mentioned previously, that person was my mother. The role of the Advocate, the Caretaker, and the Benefactor in the recovery of a Lyme victim is often what it takes to get them the right help. A friend, family member or a loved one often plays this role, sometimes, all three roles, and is often essential for the support needed during the recovery period. Should it become necessary that you need help getting help, approach someone you can trust, and rely on their judgment to get you where you need to be. I had to rely on family members and friends completely during my 44 months of antibiotic treatment, as some of even the most basic tasks were impossible.

Persistence and sheer determination are essential during treatment. After establishing an antibiotic protocol that is effective, maintaining a persistent and consistent course for the duration required to rid the body of the disease, for as long as it takes, is essential to be cured. A stubborn countenance is helpful in these circumstances. It will test your resolve, your endurance, and your will. I took 400mg of Biaxin, 200mg of Plaquenil, and 400mg of Doxycycline for forty-four months before the symptoms finally subsided and recall only one time when I forgot to take it—NYE 2010. The *only* thing I was determined to do was to keep taking that protocol regularly and consistently. That determination and consistency got me through to the end.

The role of "supplements"—diet, vitamins, natural herbs, and pharmaceuticals—all play a big role in your ability to withstand the excruciating symptoms of recovery. Medication to control pain, anxiety and depression are often essential. They are our "temporary friends" while we endure the course of treatment. I took Lyrica for widespread pain, Clonazepam for severe anxiety and sleeplessness, and Prozac for depression, and these were absolutely necessary for me to withstand the relentless symptoms of treatment. There were many times I resisted these temporary helpers, but it was always at the expense of my own unnecessary agony. There is no advantage to being resistant to taking these supplements—they are necessary, but temporary. I am now completely free of all these medications, including the antibiotics.

For most, money is an issue with Lyme treatment, even if you have more money than most. Health insurers, like most doctors, do not recognize Lyme as a legitimate condition for treatment. For me personally, Lyme disease consumed everything and eventually lead to divorce, foreclosure and bankruptcy. Once the downward spiral began, the dominoes fell and there seemed to be no stopping it. But the single largest cost was the permanent inability to earn income. Robbed of the ability to recover financially is not just a huge setback, it is a devastating personal ordeal. Adjustments to a new life are just the beginning of the end of the first ordeal. Even for the few that emerge victorious over the onslaughts of the disease coming out of the Swamp, often it carries the additional burden of a lifetime of permanent disabilities. To recover and maintain an improved quality of life that will never be what it was frequently requires drastic changes to lifestyle, behavior and personality.

As doctors and insurance do not recognize Lyme as a legitimate disability, obtaining Social Security Disability benefits for the crippling effects of Lyme are systematically denied. In order to qualify for Social Security disability, the patient must find a "specialist" that will properly misdiagnose their condition under the mantle of one or more of the many neuro-conditions that will qualify as a *legitimate disability.* Even then, the process for qualifying presents another set of hurdles that will take up to two years for a final decision. The automatic response from the Social Security Administration, except in extreme cases involving pending cases of certain death, is to routinely deny the first claim. This requires more doctor visits to the "specialist(s)" who are paid to mistreat you further under their care, costing precious time and money while the patient spirals further down into the Lyme abyss.

It is almost as if the entire process is setup to guarantee that you will become permanently disabled.

Nearly *everything* about the process seems designed to make you fail.

Often the lack of a Caretaker, Advocate and/or Benefactor presents huge obstacles for many, if not most, against the labyrinth of roadblocks, dead ends and other setbacks so characteristic of the journey. When I finally prevailed with Social Security Disability, I had already been in treatment for over six months. Then, under the watchful eye of a Caretaker, I also leaned on my parents for financial support during that time, as I was effectually incompetent to do just about anything. I was very fortunate indeed to have this network of support. These advantages might at first seem trite or insignificant, but they add up to a defensive strategy against the bewildering resistance and utter nonsense encountered in the medical community.

By the time most Lyme victims stagger, crawl or are otherwise dragged by someone else into the office of a Lyme-literate doctor, their ability to care for themselves is severely diminished. In fact, everything about the journey of the Lymer seems to be instituted in direct contrast to their getting well. But, despite the obstacles and the controversy over whether chronic Lyme disease exists, many have been cured with long-term antibiotic treatment. The medical community, backed by the CDC and the IDSA and their minions, continue to deny this. Why?

1) It would be an admission that they are wrong and have been wrong for decades;

2) It would expose their complicity in suppressing this information and expose them to legal action;

3) It protects large numbers of so-called "specialists" who are making enormous sums of money by deliberately *perpetuating* illnesses instead of *curing* them.

Deliberately keeping people sick through attempts to deceive the public would be *willful negligence and malpractice on a colossal scale.* With so much to lose, not just their reputation, but all their power and most of all, their money. To admit that persistent chronic Lyme exists would in effect expose them to a liability beyond comprehension. This is yet the tip of the iceberg in the big picture.

Once held as the "Great Imitator," we know now that this myth is giving way to the reality that chronic Lyme is actually *the "Great Initiator"* and the source of the many neurological and psychiatric illnesses. Meanwhile, they continue to protect their own interests at the expense, suffering and misery of millions. The controversy is no longer about whether chronic Lyme exists, it is about why the CDC, FDA and the IDSA continue to subvert the truth about this tragic and largely preventable epidemic."

Don't rule out Lyme until Lyme has been ruled out!

As recovery continued to restore life back to and beyond, it became ever more obvious that the fraud of Lyme disease was continuing rampantly throughout our society and across the globe. Nearly all nations of the world are involved. Virtually no one has escaped the impact. The medical community continues to misdirect attention to anything and everything possible *except* the one thing they do not want you to see.

The Lyme-crime con-game with all of its players, purveyors and victims unabatedly and unabashedly promote all sorts of phony fixes, medical procedures, pharmaceutical treatments, false diagnoses, and deliberate attempts to mislead and mis-inform.

Doctors and insurers alike are quite willing to charge for expensive medical procedures and bogus treatments that further delay the correct diagnosis. Rather than treat patients with relatively less expensive antibiotic treatment, they promote long-term chronic disease care that they claim there is no cure for. Even replacing knees, joints, and shoulders with artificial parts; there seems no limit to what they will prescribe except the one thing that has proven to work.

Ever more apparent to the few who have survived to thrive once again, the chorus of voices raised in a growing crescendo describe more than feigned ignorance. Response to this deliberate denial has unleashed an avalanche of awareness campaigns to raise the flag and warn the public. Released video presentations of the highly acclaimed "*Under Our Skin*" and the sequel "*Emergence*" are two examples of this. Meanwhile, as the campaign for awareness continues, the CDC, FDA, IDSA and the NIH continue their own self-protection campaign.

We have been taught since birth to believe what we are told. Unfortunately, this is not always in our own best interest. What we are told and what we believe can produce conflicts of interest when those who would gain personally highlight *their* best interests at the expense of others. This is what we are experiencing at the hands of modern medicine today. We accept what we are being told is true in the blind-faith that those entrusted with our health and well-being are doing so out of the goodness of their heart. This is not the case. Where money has such power, the temptation becomes too great to resist. Yet as with overcoming all such struggles, it is the individual who must decide what is best for themselves.

This concept is illustrated in the video presentation "*Don't Rule Out Lyme Until Lyme Has Been Ruled Out*!" released on the *Lymester* on February 22, 2016. It attempts to describe the human tendency to believe what we are told, based upon what we want to hear. Some seek reassurance that what they are being told is true over accepting the reality of its contrary. This could be the single-most important issue and yet the subtlest crux of the Lyme debacle.

[*The Lymester—2/22/16*] "There are two kinds of people when it comes to medical care—those who truly desire to know the truth about their diagnosis and condition, and those who seek reassurance that what they *believe* they are being told is the truth. This is certainly the case with those afflicted with Lyme. Often, we are needless victims of the latter, because we have been taught since birth to trust our doctor's knowledge, opinion and advice. But even doctors reside in one of the two camps of medical care—those who dare to consider that perhaps what they have been taught in medical school may not be the "truth, the whole truth, and nothing but the truth," and those that accept dogmatically only what they have been taught, and not to question it. This rule applies to both conventional doctors, as in your typical family practitioners, and the so-called "specialists," and to a large degree alternative holistic doctors as well. In 99.9% of these cases, well intentioned doctors believe they are doing their best to provide the best care possible to their patients. However, this has absolutely nothing to do with the accuracy of diagnosis when it comes to Lyme disease, as most practitioners are conditioned to recommend treatment of symptoms and their effects, and not cure causes. Often seen is the endless cycle of those who blindly follow the conventional path, with no eyes to see and no ears to hear, but for a small percentage of those who seemingly by Fate alone find the true cause, and even more narrowly, find the path to the cure. To break this cycle is to become knowledgeable, as has been said, knowledge is power. For those who have the knowledge, it is not their responsibility to force other people into "believing" something different from what they are being told, but merely to hold the light on the path for those who have the desire, and the Will to seek real knowledge instead of emotional reactions reflecting their doctors "belief."

The inherent problem that underlies the lack of desire and will to find real knowledge is the disease itself. Unlike other chronic diseases like heart disease and cancer, where the patient is earnestly trying to find out for sure, the Lyme victim often lacks the reason and the will to find out about their condition when it is presented as possibly Lyme. The common excuses are "Well, I don't recall being bitten by a tick," or even if they have, "I never got the bulls-eye rash," or "I've been told that it can't be Lyme because of where I live," or "I've been told that it is something else." These are the typical excuses that a Lymer will roll out in defense of their lack of desire or will to find out. ALL doctors, but for the very few Lyme-literate doctors, remain unaware that Lyme and the related co-infections are transmitted not only from tick bites from infected ticks, but through the public blood supply, or passed to the unborn child from an infected mother, or transmitted as a sexually transmitted disease (STD). And conventional medicine is all too willing to convince you of a brand of disease that they can continue to treat indefinitely without ever seeking an actual cause and cure, which would be our so-called "chronic diseases" that they claim "there is no known cure" for. This continued perpetuation of the ignorance of Lyme disease, it's widespread permeating of the population, and the resultant suffering in terms of cost and misery, is staggering.

Mainly through denial, the Lyme victim seeks to justify their disease by belief in their doctor's misdiagnosis, seeking reassurance that their doctor is correct, meanwhile earnestly and sometimes militantly defending this position against anything to do with considering Lyme as the culprit. The main reason for this is that Lyme is primarily a neuro-psychiatric condition that affects the central nervous system, including the brain where the seat of reason and intelligence resides. When reason and logic have become disabled, the patient is no longer capable of the kind of objective judgment that otherwise might occur to a cancer or heart disease patient. The militant defiance to anything to do with Lyme could be a curious indicator of the disease, where reason and logic have taken flight. When the patients decision-making ability doesn't make sense, look for Lyme."

PART 5

Debunking Popular Myths about Lyme Disease

Is Borrelia the Perfect Man-Made "Stealth Pathogen?"

"The questions when and how the infection took place are even quite irrelevant to his present condition. Even the most accurate knowledge of the previous history cannot cure tuberculosis. And the same holds true for [Lyme]."
—Carl Jung

Much debate and controversy has been stirred up over whether the Borrelia spirochete may have been genetically modified in the post-WWII labs of bio-warfare. The notorious Plum Island lab off the coast of Long Island, New York made famous in Nelson Melville's book "*Plum Island*" is testament to the possibility the disease could have originated there. Other documentation of syphilis combined with Borrelia-type bacteria during the late 1950's also suggest the same possibility. The infamous report known as *LAB-257* documents the advances of microbiology to secure bio-warfare agents in the ongoing effort to potentially destroy ourselves as well as our enemies.

Other documented sources which describe experiments with syphilis (another spirochetal organism) genetically combined or spliced with Borrelia as early as the early 1950's, suggests that the WWII *Paperclip* efforts to import German Nazi bio-technology were well underway. By the 1960's, under the direction of Eric Traub, a well-known Nazi infectious disease scientist specializing in bacterium and viruses, was experimenting with ticks on the very eve of the first diagnosed cases of Lyme disease.

Though it is unlikely that we will ever know whether the disease was released intentionally or not, it does suggest that the organism responsible for the outbreak could be determined as one genetically designed to evade or disable the immune system.

Some evidence of this is suggested in current bio-research of the Borrelia organism, where the most advanced biologist researchers are baffled at the complexity and stealth-like characteristics by which it thrives unimpeded by natural defenses. This further suggests why long-term antibiotic treatment is favored over natural remedies, as there is of yet no known substance in nature that can effectively cure Borrelia. This further suggests the organism is a creation of science and not of nature. What may be an entirely appropriate comment about why long-term antibiotic treatment seems to work best when compared to natural remedies with regards to Borrelia:

"It takes science to undo what science has created."

Borreliosis Basics: the Facts Behind the Science

[August 26, 2014] Borreliosis is a multi-system disease caused by a spirochetal bacterium (parasite). A spirochete is a spiral-shaped parasite with a unique mechanism for movement that features a bundle of tail-like "flagella" which reside inside the cell wall.

Borreliosis is transmitted primarily through the bite of an infected tick, but also may be transmitted by insect vectors, in utero to an unborn fetus, (says Yale), and possibly via sexual intercourse. If not treated immediately with antibiotics, the infection can persist for years and cause symptoms often diagnosed as neurological diseases such as MS, Lupus, cancer, Chronic Fatigue, Myalgic Encephalomyelitis, ALS (Lou Gehrig's Disease) and Alzheimer's, according to IDSA and the CDC. Thus, borreliosis is commonly referred to as "The Great Imitator" or "New Great Imitator."

Borreliae parasites have the ability to shed (bleb off) their outer membrane lipoproteins to evade detection by the immune system in a mechanism commonly known as antigenic variation. These lipoproteins are called "outer surface proteins" (OspA) and "variable major proteins" (Vmp). In layman's terms, the blebbing, or shedding, of OspA by the borreliae parasite sends the immune system after the OspA, allowing the spirochete to hide from immune attack and persist in the host.

Additionally, several of these outer surface lipoproteins, such as OspA (the Lyme "vaccine"), are TLR-2 agonists or fungal antigens, meaning they essentially disable the immune system. They do this by way of tolerance to other fungal antigens (TLR2s) as well as tolerance to other antigen types, managed by other TLRs.

See this report: "Because IRAK1 is required for TLR7/9-induced IFN-I production, we propose that TLR2 signaling induces rapid depletion of IRAK1, which impairs IFN-I induction by TLR7/9. This novel mechanism, whereby TLR2 inhibits IFN-I induction by TLR7/9, may shape immune responses to microbes that express ligands for both TLR2 and TLR7/TLR9, or responses to bacteria/virus coinfection." *http://www.ncbi.nlm.nih.gov/pubmed/22227568*

Exposure to shed borrelial lipoproteins causes fungal tolerance in the blood and the inability to get rid of mycoplasma/eperythrozoons from the blood, especially from the red blood cells (which causes fatigue). Also, there is cross-tolerance to TLR4 agonists from constant TLR2-agonism of shed borrelial antigens like OspA and vice-versa. (This is in the literature, so help yourself.) This creates an environment where opportunistic infections can thrive and cause chronic, disabling disease. TLR2-agonist tolerance apparently reactivates latent herpes viruses, particularly Epstein Barr Virus (EBV). (Reactivation occurs thru IL-10, and the inhibition of apoptosis of OspA or EBV infected cells, the mechanism shown above re TLR2-signaling and the inhibition of IFN-I, and perhaps other unknown mechanisms.)

Chronic EBV is probably the main driver of all these New Great and Great Imitator diseases.

There is no misery greater than surviving when the will to do so no longer exists. The fact that this is not air-borne tells us something—that this is not intended as a quick demise, but a slow misery worse than death itself. The Borrelia pathogen seems to be designed precisely for this purpose. Rather than a relatively quick 24-72 hour ordeal that the Black Plague, typhus, the Spanish influenza, Ebola and the other hemophlagiac viruses deliver, the stealth pathogen of the Borrelia bacterium delivers a slow, agonizing, crippling effect designed to disable the immune system and promote the advancement of other natural pathogens, but not kill outright. This is similar to the emergence of AIDS and the Gulf-war Syndrome known as post-traumatic-stress-disorder (PTSD). What might take a deadly virus several days to accomplish takes several decades with the Borrelia bacterium. Limited by the four modes of transmission, the parasite can remain, for the most part, undetected and maintain its stealth nature. This permits the "creep" of the disease to proliferate mostly undetected until when finally discovered, it is virtually too late for the victim.

The malady common to ex-military soldiers of the Gulf War under President George W. Bush, Sr. referred to as "Gulf-War Syndrome" is remarkably similar to the effects of Lyme disease. Chronic fatigue and degenerative neuro-disorders commonly known as Post Traumatic Stress Disorder (PTSD) suggest a similar cause or infectious disease origin. Some experts have argued that the common bacteria known as mycoplasma may play a role, as it is also suspect in vaccines and as possible sources of autism. The blatant lack of investigation and the intentional secrecy behind the research of these organisms point to a concerted effort on the part of the government and the military to suppress information about them, and suggests fear on their part of releasing information that might expose any possible hint of a deliberate conspiracy about Lyme disease.

Counter to the investigative efforts of biological research, many micro-biologists have disappeared under mysterious circumstances in the past several decades. The mycoplasma bacterial organism has since been patented by the US government. Trying to find *any* general information about *mycoplasma* is nearly impossible. It seems the name itself is a carefully guarded secret.

Perhaps what we collectively fear most is knowing the truth. There is an eerie parallel to the stealthy advance of the predatory nature of Lyme disease and the predatory nature of our society.

Change is the very essence of the activity that comprises the material world, and yet all forms of our current institutions are influenced to stop, arrest, prevent or control this change. Psychologist Erich Fromm explains that our contemporary view of human civilization is born in the modern age of science and technology, begun in the late 19th century and applied to industrial society as a form of psychological manipulation and human engineering:

> *"The contemporary vision, however, is that of unlimited consumption and unlimited control over nature. Men are fired by the dream that one day they will completely control nature*

and thus be like God; why should there by anything in *__human__* *nature that cannot be controlled?"*

The preservation of the "status quo" of civilization is the Holy Grail of all political institutions; to prevent or control change and preserve its power at all times. This is often invoked in the name of the "greatest good" by way of distraction and deception. It appeals to the primal emotional subconscious to evoke fear of change and manipulates human desire for safety and freedom from fear, real or imagined.

There exists an eerie parallel between "intentional suffering" and Lyme disease, as with the other plagues of the past. Our attempts to control nature have a retaliatory effect on our ability to thrive in that world without self-inflicted suffering. The tendency to want to explain this phenomenon as a type of instinctual determinism, that self-inflicted suffering is an unchangeable part of human nature is refuted by Fromm, but clearly holds its own with some of Fromm's contemporaries. Fromm explains by quoting R. Waelder's view of a "new instinctivism" in human affairs due to our attempts to manipulate and exploit our environment:

> *"As I have pointed out, one reason for this is the sense of fear and hopelessness that pervades many people because of the ever-increasing dangers and that nothing is done to avert them. Many who had faith in progress and had hoped for basic changes in man's fate, instead of carefully analyzing the social process which led to their disillusionment, are taking refuge in the explanation that man's nature must be responsible for this failure. Finally, there are the personal and political biases of the authors who become spokesman for the new instinctivism… no believer in the fundamental goodness of man and in the exclusive responsibility of external causes of human suffering could help being disturbed by a theory of an instinct of destruction or a death instinct. For if this theory is true, potentialities for conflict and for suffering are inherent in human affairs, and attempts to abolish or mitigate suffering appear to be, if not hopeless undertakings, at least far more complicated ones than the social revolutionaries had fancied them to be."*

Fromm refutes this observation, and goes on to demonstrate human suffering is not instinctual, but rooted in our "human character", as a result of being in the world of Nature:

> *"...that destructiveness and cruelty [the origins of suffering] are not instinctual drives, but passions rooted in the total existence of man. They are one of the ways to make sense of life; they are by their very nature rooted in the "human condition." The main error of the instinctivists is to have confused the two kinds of drives; those rooted in the instinct, and those rooted in character."*

The possibility that human behavior is *learned*, acquired culturally as the root cause of our own suffering, is still largely ignored and dismissed by modern science. The consequences of blind ambition to control nature by the promise of science, in exchange for economic advantage over unmitigated materialist consumption, are beginning to show their effects. The consumption model depends exclusively on obedience and submission of the individual to its doctrine.

> *[Fromm] "...gigantic centralized enterprises and its capacity to provide the workers with amusements and bread, is able to maintain control by psychological manipulation and human engineering. It needs a man who is very malleable and easily influenced, rather than those whose "instincts" are controlled by fears or authority."*

Small wonder that advances in experimentation with microbes, viruses, bacteria and compromised insects have been engineered in government bio-labs since WWII and earlier. What better way to control a population than to disable, cripple the will, the ability to think on their own, and the ability to defend themselves.

Counter-intuitive to everything we have been told and taught, this theory has only just begun to be explored and requires further examination. Our undivided attention and objective critical analysis of this phenomena is *key to our survival*. This is a very uncomfortable subject for most people.

What is this most perplexing phenomena of self-destructiveness that plagues humanity in every generation, in every epoch of civilization and society? Is it not enough that we define and defend ourselves against forces inherent in the natural world for survival? The pattern suggests that we are *created* to suffer. When suffering is alleviated by our dominance over the forces of nature by and the efforts of "civilization," it seems we then prey upon ourselves to counterbalance nature and exact the required debt of suffering. It's as if this price of suffering must be paid one way or the other, either from the external forces of nature, or self-inflicted in the absence of natural adversity. *We* become are our own worst enemy.

Five Myths about Lyme Disease and "The Lie Too Big to Admit."

Current myths and superstitions about Lyme are generally not well documented. There remains a lack of awareness of these, despite some authors and researchers claiming the contrary. This is especially true for the medical community, who appears to be always last to recognize and accept the advances of medical science. However, they are slowly and reluctantly acknowledging the latest advances in research, uncovering evidence of a "lie too big to admit."

Despite slow acceptance of these facts emerging in greater frequency and urgency, the nay-sayers continue to protect increasingly untenable positions. At stake are power, money and a tenacious defense of reputations based upon these myths. Increasingly, the overwhelming evidence of the truth behind Lyme will eventually expose the deniers. Why so many innocent victims must suffer is perhaps beyond our comprehension or ability to answer, but those who stand for a better world make it possible.

As is commonly understood about truth, it cannot be suppressed and denied forever. But, whether we are the cause of it or otherwise is irrelevant to those who suffer. It is up to each of us to face our own truth, to overcome self-denial, ignorance and self-deception. The ability to expose the culprits, hold them accountable, and seek reparations and corrections that will promote life, *and not death*, will be found when we have the courage to face our own reflection.

As we have seen in the stealthy progression of Lyme for nearly half a century now, the tide is turning in the opposite direction. The many myths, superstitions and outright lies about this plague are becoming self-evident. Attempts to suppress and deny the very existence of the disease, and the "lie too big to admit," continues to be exposed from every corner. As truth is always the last to prevail, it will set us free, but not from what was endured to expose it.

Myth #1: Lyme as the "Great Imitator"

Largest of the Lyme myths is the "Great Imitator," the notion that

Lyme mimics so-called chronic diseases purported to have no known cure. We have seen the medical community for decades now describe how the persistence of Lyme *mimics* symptoms of the many chronic illnesses that currently plague human society. Evidence continues to reveal the contrary—that Lyme presents as the *source or origin* of these afflictions. Trust and respect for modern medicine continues to steadily erode due to the contrariness of the evidence.

Clearly we can see now that in actuality Lyme disease and its related co-infections are the "*Great Originator*" of modern chronic illness.

Seen consistently in the emergence of this modern plague are the characteristics of a single source of an undetected origin, from which neurological, psychological, psychiatric and muscular-skeletal maladies have sprung.

This rising tide of mysterious illnesses, complicated with myriads of changing and migrating symptoms, is largely indicative of a single source such as Lyme and it's related co-infections. A common origin, a single source for the majority of related illnesses has increased in frequency and severity amongst all age groups. Though increasingly the evidence suggests that this is the case, it certainly does not suggest that *all* these modern afflictions are caused by a single source, but instead a high *probability there is a common source* for a large majority of them. It does not require a medical degree or a genius to connect the dots.

Myth #2: Lyme comes from an infected tick.

As we know today, there are **four known modes** of transmission.

1) The bite of an infected tick;

2) From sexual contact with an infected individual;

3) Passed to the unborn fetus from mothers who are infected;

4) Spread through the public blood supply through infected blood donors.

The myth about ticks as the single-source of Lyme is over. Overwhelming new evidence to the contrary can no longer be denied. Whether ticks remain as the *primary* source of infections is debatable. New evidence of the Borrelia spirochete transmitted sexually perhaps as easily as the syphilis spirochete may by far be the largest source of dissemination of the disease. The medical community's stand on this new evidence is indicative of how far denial has gone. The inevitable truth of this new evidence is stealthily revealing itself to our waking consciousness.

Myth #3: Lyme infection typically presents with a bull's eye rash.

This is not true. The infamous "bull's eye rash" often required to prove the predominant evidence of the Lyme spirochete occurs in a small minority of cases resulting from a tick bite. To rely on this clinical observation for beginning antibiotic treatment is like waiting for a patient's head to explode before treating them for meningitis. Physicians who decline treatment at the earliest possible stages of Lyme and wait for further symptoms to develop before administering known cures is not only in violation of the Hippocratic Oath, but complicit in willful negligence and malpractice. There is simply no excuse for this practice anymore.

Myth #4: Lyme is hard to get and easy to cure.

This is a lie. Nothing could be further from the truth. We have known for *years* that this is not the case. Persistence of the bacterium after minimal duration of treatment with antibiotics is widely known and accepted, and there is no excuse for this type of misinformation. Deliberately misleading the public about the fact that Lyme is *not* necessarily cured simply with a maximum of a 3-30 day period of antibiotic treatment is all about protection for perpetrators of known lies.

Myth #5: There is no cure for advanced late-stage Lyme.

Popular literature, articles and on-line tutorials about this subject are most of the time not intentionally misleading, but mis-informed. Most of the severely afflicted fail in treatment from lack of *duration* in their antibiotic treatment. When months and years roll by with no change in their symptoms, the inclination to give up treatment is understandable. Though it is now understood that the cure is more of a long-distance run than a sprint to the finish line, it is *not* yet understood why the duration of long-term antibiotic treatment works. It may have something to do with the reproductive cycles of the Borrelia organism, consistently exposed to an antibiotic environment over time. Future research of these characteristics will eventually reveal the nature of its stubborn subsistence, resistance to the treatment and how it damages the immune system. In time, experience will eventually reveal the truth that a cure is possible, as can already be seen by the testimonials of those who have experienced and witnessed a cure. Tainted research designed to support and protect the positions of medical professionals cannot stand indefinitely.

This comes to the greatest myth about modern medicine:

"First do no harm."

Personally, this was the hardest one to come to understand and finally give up. The ignorance on the part of modern medicine is easier to understand, but *denial*? That was difficult to accept. Where money is involved in health-care, this will always take precedence over actual well-being. There is no profit motive in well-being when so much more money can be made from perpetuating disease. This is evidenced in the many government and health agencies that are purported to exist for the benefit of the patient. This is simply not the case. Most evidence points to the opposite.

We have been led to believe that the Hippocratic Oath "first do no harm", taken by the medical professionals we place our trust in, would *never* have to be questioned. Until now, it has become the "lie too big to admit."

Perpetuating the Veil of Ignorance and Denial

"The Emperor has no clothes" has never been more apparent than in this current dystopia of corporate medicine. The veil of denial is getting thin indeed. In fact, it is nearly transparent. Never has desperation for intervention and interference on such an incredulous scale ever been proposed. The obvious fact of the blind-leading-the-blind has never been more apparent. And yet, the FDA, CDC and IDSA continue to stand by the preposterous claim that post-treatment Lyme disease *does not exist.* While the public still clings to illusions that these institutions were created to protect them, the medical community continues to do everything in their power to preserve their own power and protect their interests.

Protection of the Perpetrators

It is a well-known fact that the bigger the lie the more effort it takes to suppress the truth. How could science that we have been taught to believe and idolize in the 21st century betray us so willfully and so completely? Can we even identify who the real perpetrators are?

The answer is not an easy one.

By intensive inner contemplation, self-reflection takes us beyond our comfort zone where the tendency to avoid the truth is so much *easier.* Avoiding confrontation of uncomfortable truths about ourselves, as well as each other, is what our daily existence is designed for; to distract, dissuade, hide and suppress the truth about ourselves. Protecting its own vital interests, these invisible forces are working constantly to perpetuate our self-deceptions for the sake of its own existence.

This is seen constantly in the news media, advertising, and in our everyday common social dialogue. Stimulation of reaction to illusory fear followed by distractions of superficial escape and pleasure, cast over and over in "spin" that consume the viewers' day, blot out the truth and mask the real underlying issues. The endless chatter of breaking news, politicians, their pundits and paid advertisers constantly manipulate decision-making at the sub-conscious level and lull us into the daydream that things are okay, that we are safe from purported dangers, the Status Quo is preserved at all costs.

This parasitic form of government and control is a reflection of our belief in it. It dominates our thinking, our social and political institutions, and our belief systems in science and evolution.

The Crisis of Modern Science in Medicine

"We thus come to those ultimate questions: Whence does consciousness come? What is the psyche? And at this point all science ends."
—Carl Jung in "Modern Man in Search of a Soul"

Even in our observations and reflections of this phenomena, we seem unable, or *unwilling*, to confront these self-inflicted causes. We continue to seek foreign enemies as a scapegoat, a projection of our fears and self-delusions, when we already *have* a common enemy: *ignorance* and *denial*. This two-headed monster compromises our human condition. Carefully guarded and hidden, this self-deception is of our own making and by our own choice.

We have been taught to believe our social and cultural institutions protect us from unseen and unpredictable outside forces, over which we have little or no control. Hidden, lurking beneath the surface of consciousness, a primal *fear* of our external nature causes human behavior to prey upon itself.

Knowledge of the physical world has led to advances in technology and arguably has presented many effective creature comforts as it's reward. But at what price? It has done *nothing* to enhance our understanding of our spiritual origins, the nature of man, or our existential dilemma of "being in the world" of nature. Nor have there been significant improvements in our overall human condition of perpetual war, famine, poverty and disease. The failure of the material sciences to deliver understanding of our reason and purpose in the world is in itself evidence to the contrary. Why is it that science, with its prowess in technological advancement, has produced new and better ways to kill on a *massive* scale but not delivered on promoting peace? Why is the focus of science on economic systems based on justifications for "self-defense" from fabricated external threats of dubious origins? Are these limits, of what reason and science have to offer, protection from false fear based upon the rewards of "comfort" and the distractions of entertainment?

Clearly the advances of the physical sciences since the 18th century in medicine, engineering, industry, astronomy, biology, etc., as well as innovations of technology in the 19th and 20th century, have served humanity's interests and needs in the form of creature comforts. Proud recognition, adulation and idolatry that was once reserved for the divine soul are now donned upon the wave of modern materialism emerging from the earlier days of the Renaissance, and the subsequent revolution of the physical sciences which crested in the 20th century. Yet, the rewards of physical comfort and genuine human advancement seem to be hijacked at every step, marred by violence, hatred and the chaos of two world wars. The dominance of science over the boundaries of human consciousness is maintained in all areas and activities of human society and culture in the name of the *status quo*.

Eastern philosopher Alan Watt's in his book "*Behold the Spirit*" discusses the role of science as a reflection of maturity of the human species, and whether or not it has developed fruit from union with the human spirit. Consequences of conformity to immoral impulses becomes a "curse upon the face of the earth" when science is focused on personal gain over others:

> *"It is a fruit of union that men should desire to heal the sick to prolong life and health. It is a fruit of union that they should study the secrets of nature and develop sciences and skills to this end. But when these goals are pursued for their own sake, when their original impulse and their final end are forgotten*

> *and untaught, the power of healing becomes a power of destruction. It is a fruit of union that men should study agriculture and engineering to feed the hungry and clothe the naked, but when the object of production becomes profit alone, the moral impulse has failed in its object and become positively immoral."*

Difficult, perhaps, to accept but not to understand, there is no joy, happiness, rest, laughter or comfort ever given or accepted without infliction of some form of misery and suffering in return. Karma has its way of divvying out payment for transgressions committed by the spirit at the expense of the soul. There are two forms of payment: suffering or atonement. Acts of virtue—charity, compassion, mercy, empathy, tolerance, forbearance, love—are expressions of the divine. Acts committed on behalf of the ego—the seven deadly sins—are paid in *suffering*.

Dostoevski quotes:

> *"Suffering is not only profoundly inherent in man, but it is the sole cause of the awakening of conscious thought."*

Also, in the form of Buddha as the "awakened one" according to Dane Rudhyar, overcoming human suffering is a function of awareness:

> *"No man can become truly and actually 'human' save by reaching a state of maximum clarity and wakefulness. And this state is symbolized in Asia by the figure of the Buddha, the Awakened, the Illumined, the absolutely Clear One. In him humanity came to a condition of total and unqualified acceptance of all human experience, to a state of undisturbed wakefulness and lucidity, free from illusion, glamor and uncertainty. He dared to face facts, all the facts. He dared to contain all reality known to man—to include in his clear consciousness the experience of hell as well as of heaven. And, in him, every experience a human being ever lived anywhere became significant. He 'shaped' all experiences unto the likeness of his all-inclusive self-hood; for his being had become a vessel, container of all. Thus, he overcame suffering."*

Science is yet to prove our relationship to the divine as alchemy did prior to our modern Age of Reason, yet recent discoveries in quantum physics suggests that our universe is an all-connected, all pervasive vibratory substance, a vibrant living being. Our role in nature is being redefined by this knowledge as rapidly as we race against inevitable self-destruction. And yet the question remains—if we are to *overcome* suffering, how? Or, are we to *accept* suffering and thereby overcome it through this acceptance? This answer is ultimately *both*. Or neither.

PART 6

Affliction of The Spirit: The Diabolical Side of Lyme Disease

"Thus, I considered all my activities which my hands had done and the labor which I had exerted, and behold all was vanity and striving after wind and there was no profit under the sun."
—Ecclesiastes 2:11

A most perplexing observation amongst some of the afflicted is an astonishing resistance to becoming well again. Some of the severely compromised are confronted with the crippling inability to exercise the human faculties of reason and the will, which leaves them with few choices but emotional reactions to the feeling of being trapped. An incomprehensible inability or unwillingness to help themselves takes over, despite numerous attempts by concerned friends, family members and doctors. The Lyme victim seems stubbornly bent on succumbing to hopelessness and their own self-destruction. Seemingly determined to find ways to deny or refuse help, they consistently subvert their own and others attempts to assist in deliberate acts of self-sabotage.

A stubborn, tenacious part of the will takes over and inexplicably turns against itself. Even when the Lyme victim sees the inevitable train wreck coming, they purposely and deliberately dodge any attempt to derail the process. Attempts to help are systemically ignored or dismissed and sometimes even violently rejected. As symptoms worsen, admonishments seem to further fortify the will against itself in a downward spiral of self-destruction. It is most unfortunate that it finally comes to this point before the Lymer seeks help, when others have given up trying and the possibility of a journey back seems most unlikely.

When help finally arrives, it can often seem too late. Depersonalizing the self, it often manifests psychiatric conditions of personality and/or identity disorders, depression, bi-polar disorder, schizophrenia, etc. Its effects on behavior and character can be dramatic, sometimes changing the character or personality of its victim into wholly other identities. *"He's not the same anymore"* is a frequent assessment. Having given up any thought of hope or recovery, the Lymer often refuses treatment or doing anything that would alter or reverse the progress of the disease. This form of resignation that surrenders the victim to the predator, is what is described here as "diabolical."

It is a small wonder the Lyme victim lapses into despair and depression. The effects and consequences of refusing or rejecting treatment are seen in the decline of the spirit. Often everything previously obtained is lost—money, possessions, careers—but most of all the ability to do even simple things. Being unable to work or contribute is difficult beyond measure, especially for experienced givers who now must be receivers. Absent are the friends whom we used to enjoy doing things with. Even those closest to us, our family members, sometimes do not recognize or refuse to acknowledge Lyme as a possibility for what appears as lackadaisical loafing, laziness, hypochondria or malingering types of behavior. Profound and tragic is the effect on those who, of no fault of their own, cannot defend themselves against these accusations.

The loss of physical and mental strength is reflected deeply in the spirit, which suffers equally to the body; perhaps greater. Compound this with departure of friends and acquaintances with whom one no longer interacts with and it compares to victims of stroke or dementia. The effects are similar. The loss of hope is all too familiar for those robbed of so much, and with so little to look forward to. Why does the Lyme victim permit these conditions to persist even when they know how they are produced? It is perplexing that those who need help the most are defiant in their efforts to refuse it. Do some Lyme victims affix blame on themselves for their fate? Do some of those who suffer in some circumstances feel they deserve their fate?

As absurd as this sounds, the source of affliction appears self-driven, a form of self-punishment endured while intentionally resisting interference by others. The sheer indifference the Lyme victim can show towards their own recovery, or worse, the *deliberate* sabotage of their own health appears as a severe form of intentional self-infliction. The onlooker must ask whether there is something to this. Ignoring what at first seems ridiculous or unthinkable is a major obstacle to understanding this improbable phenomena.

The fear engendered by the Lyme victim produces an insidious form of paralysis, rendering the will unable to act. As the onset of the disease attacks the neocortex, the amygdala and the hypothalamus parts of the brain tissue, thinking and emotional processes become increasingly impaired, giving rise to irrational behavior, impulsive reactions and poor judgment. Often a malignant form of "fight or flight" syndrome develops from over-stimulation of the instinct for self-preservation. The struggle for survival overwhelms the senses in a semi-permanent form of Post-Traumatic Stress Disorder (PTSD) or "chronic anxiety."

Often seen in the charade of modern chronic illnesses of which Lyme is the source, these symptoms are frequently misdiagnosed as mental illness. The well-meaning psychologist or psychiatrist, or in the office of chronic disease "specialists"—the neurologist, rheumatologist, etc.—these otherwise well-meaning doctors are also victims of this debacle. Caught in the web of money and the tendency to emphasize treatment of symptoms while ignoring causes pushes the dilemma further up the pyramid where professors of medical schools and universities are taught and pass down the same doctrine—ignore the *causes* and treat the *symptoms*. The entire medical community begins to emerge as an upside-down and backward system stacked, intentionally or otherwise, against the individual sufferer, actually compromising the very support structure the patient so desperately needs!

Clearly self-evident now there is something essentially mysterious about the nature of how this illness is being handled, and specifically so with the current Lyme epidemic. With the CDC now forced to admit to overwhelming evidence of over 300,000 new cases per year, suppression of the truth about Lyme and the oppression of its victims reveals a monstrous truth.

As incredulous as this sounds, a better explanation behind the twisted intent characterizing this insidious disease has not been forthcoming. This is not a mistake, it is *intentional*. And, as long as these forces are successful at keeping us from understanding this, the predatory-parasitic model is maintained. These behaviors cannot persist without its consequences: war, famine, poverty and *disease*.

The cure we so desperately seek is ultimately not found in the external world, as we have been led to believe. Antibiotics, vaccines, diet, will do little to stem the rising tide and the wake of misery that follows without applying them first to the causes. The answers and solutions we seek are first nurtured *within our own souls*. The values reflected in the external world are returned to us from without as manifestations of our collective human consciousness. Therein resides the real source of both the cause and the cure. The permanent solution to this problem will not be found in the world of medicine, politics and science, but first in the recognition of its actual source—*us*.

As Jung explains:

> *"... [there is] a discovery that is very unwelcome to the science of medicine: namely, the discovery that the psyche is an aetiological or causal factor in disease."*

Within we find what we are looking for—the origin and cause of our affliction, brought onto us by us, and ultimately resolved by us.

Lyme disease is essentially a manifestation of an affliction involving the human spirit.

Until we recognize and acknowledge this, we will continue to be the source of our own descent and demise in the physical world of Lyme disease, or whatever plague follows. By first turning our focus *inwards*, through inner contemplation and introspection, the mirror of self-reflection reveals the light of hope we seek, and the beginning of the path to actual well-being.

Are <u>we</u> the source of our own suffering?

If this is possible, then it is also possible that we are the source of our own resolution from suffering.

And I set my mind to seek and explore by wisdom concerning
all that has been done under heaven.
It is a grievous task which God has given to the sons of men
to be afflicted with.

The long periods of inactivity spent staring at the ceiling, second-by-second, minute-by-minute, hour-by-hour, day-by-day, weeks, months... every second felt like an eternity in itself, and often it seemed as if it would never end, or whether it was worth it to continue. An extreme sensation of separation of mind and body emerged, the body being a "car" or chariot, a vehicle, for carrying around the mind that dwelt inside as a completely detached passenger. This excruciating feeling of duality persisted in the long hours of meditation that became necessary for coping with treatment. Not so much an exercise of will as of *necessity*, meditation provided a kind of sanctuary while enduring the long periods of time not being able to do anything else. As all other forms of enjoyment had long departed, there was nothing left to do but wait… and wait... and wait…

So, I hated life, for the work which had been done under the sun was grievous to me;
because everything is futility and striving after wind.
—Ecclesiastes 2:17

Long before this, while still a network administrator at the Merrimack Valley School District, a persistent increase in irritability became overwhelming. Every single little thing that occurred became an obstacle to overcome. As if cursed by the opposite of the Midas Touch, instead everything turned into an absolute disaster, and there seemed little or nothing that could be done about it. Due to this rising tide of constant annoyance, a pervasive incompetence began taking over everything. Murphy's Law ruled every day now, and even things that could not possibly go wrong somehow did. Beginning softly at first but repeating over and over a small voice emerged saying "don't do anything, don't do anything, don't do anything." The more the voice was suppressed and ignored, the louder it got. I would constantly question this voice saying:

"How can this be happening? Especially to the extent that it is...
It is absolutely <u>impossible</u> for this to be happening."

A counter voice in my head would query:

"What have I done to deserve this impossible thing?
And WHY?"

The incredulity of what was happening frequently descended into a kind of morbid self-deprecation, screaming in the car on the way to work for having to turn around for the briefcase—again—left behind. Then again for the phone. Then the pager… This self-directed rage was extreme, and all the psychiatrists in the world couldn't help. "It's all just in your head… It's about your *attitude*," they would tell me. "Try walking on the sunny side of the street" they would suggest. "After all, the cup is half full, right?" The downward spiral became unstoppable, as real fear crept from the back of the mind into the front. Now a constant presence in the conscious mind, while dangling over the abyss, barely hanging on by a thread, the thought arose questioning how much longer I could prevail against the inevitable demise of life itself—of complete and utter disaster.

During the previous decade, at first increasing gradually and then with greater escalation began an underlying uneasiness, a creeping form of chronic anxiety, a dreadful feeling of *running out of time*. This feeling of pending doom was barely noticeable in 1994 when graduating from Franklin Pierce College with a Bachelor of Science degree in Information Systems. But somehow a premonition of the future being eclipsed by something disastrous soon began to loom. At first, this underlying fear was tucked away in the back of the mind, and with the help of Serzone (Nefrazodone, an SSRI for depression) I forged on to the highest level of productivity yet in my career. With a family to support and dreams and goals to accomplish, these were the highest priority. There seemed no limit to ambition and the determination to overcome, or at least outrace this creeping dread, this feeling of pending doom. Onward helter-skelter into the future I went, confident that the effort to nurture this false ambition would not be doomed to failure.

I started a journal before college in 1977, later named *The Chronicles of Despair,* that records the experiences forming the basis of this story. The tone of the dialogue began to change some ten years later. By the late 1990's, the feeling of dread had increased to the point where seeking alternative ways of making a living became a real necessity. It began to look like the specter of dread had indeed been outrun. The race with this beast nipping at my heels had apparently been left in the dust. But, in spite of the many successes along the way, there was still the underlying sense of *doom*—a dread or premonition that somehow everything we valued would succumb to a catastrophe. It became pervasive, a kind of dark premonition, an ever-present darkness that threatened everything. The more I advanced on this path of success, a counter-force behind it, like the wake of a boat through the water, slowly gained speed coming close and closer threatening to capsize the boat.

Being spiritual by nature but also an ambitious sort, I was determined to not let material success leave us behind. There would certainly be more than enough. I was determined to not let it become an issue in our family.

Today, we are taught to worship and idolize the values of egoism, of self-interest over others. This is reinforced over and over in our society, taught in education and religion, reflected in our politics, economic and social policies. Financial material success is heralded as the great achievement of our times, stimulated at the instinctual level of the subconscious through advertising with emphasis on material accumulation as the way to success in life. To have more stuff than your neighbor is the mark of success; the bigger house, the more expensive car, the greener lawn. These have become the earmarks of value that we use to measure ourselves and our success against one another. The entire system is designed around these values. Despite increasing dissatisfaction with its material benefits, a world disdaining compassion and common purpose continues to emphasize comfort and protection in favor of the easy way.

Carl Jung describes the boomerang effect of this culture of condemnation and the influence of egoism:

> *"He [mankind] knows that God has brought all sorts of strange and inconceivable things to pass, and seeks in the most curious ways to enter a man's heart. He therefore senses in everything the unseen presence of the divine will.... We cannot change anything unless we accept it. Condemnation does not liberate, it oppresses. I am the oppressor of the person I condemn, not his friend and fellow-sufferer. I do not in the least mean to say that we must never pass judgment in the cases of persons whom we desire to help and improve.... And he can do this in reality only when he has already seen and accepted himself as he is. Perhaps this sounds very simple, but simple things are always the most difficult. In actual life it requires the greatest discipline to be simple, and acceptance of oneself is the essence of the moral problem and the epitome of a whole outlook upon life... the very enemy himself – that these are within me, and that I myself am the enemy that must be loved—what then?... We hide it from the world; we refuse to admit ever having met this least among the lowly in ourselves.... To accept himself in all his wretchedness is the hardest of tasks, and one which it is almost impossible to fulfill. The very thought can make us*

> *livid with fear. We therefore do not hesitate, but lightheartedly choose the complicated course of remaining in ignorance about ourselves while busying ourselves with other people and their troubles and sins. This activity lends us an air of virtue, and we thus deceive ourselves and those around us... The conflict may be between the sensual and the spiritual man, or between the ego and the shadow… This is the source of egoism, which is one of the most tangible evils of the neurotic state."*

Those who succumb to the promise and rewards of material success risk falling into the sticky tar-trap of greed, avarice, envy, jealousy, and pride; all serving the primary idol of the narcissistic lower ego-self—*vanity*.

As the disease progressed and the medications increased, it became increasingly apparent this runaway train was headed for imminent disaster, a scheduled train wreck that could not be avoided. No longer able to remember the lyrics to my own songs when performing with the band River Hill, now they had to be read prompted from a music stand. Everything touched relating to the contract with Merrimack Valley School District resulted in more hours than were available to fix. It also became increasingly difficult to follow through with evictions of non-paying tenants from the rental properties. This three-ring circus act eventually began to feel like walking a tight-rope with no safety net while juggling six-bowling balls.

As the hi-tech career crested in 2002-2003, there were increasingly periods of escape into a fantasy of leaving it all behind for Belize. As the workload piled up around my desk until it was literally falling on the floor, the escape plot revealed the horrible possibility of *letting it go*. There was nothing to stop this anymore. All that remained was the opportunity to change myself, accordingly. What seemed an overwhelming external force of events had completely rendered me helpless and hopeless, but for a desperate attempt to remake myself in some desperate way. Thus, began my new volition as "dragon-slayer," a knight with shining armor, sword and shield to vanquish the creations of my own discontent, in one last disastrous attempt to undo what I had done.

Cutting the Trees

Once there existed a set of Gothic bull-pine trees on the path out to the old family camp along the banks of the Blackwater River by our new home. Majestic and serene, they had escaped the swath of the logger chain-saws numerous times in the past and were protected by law and deed. Some of these huge trees measured over five feet thick at the base and would easily take 3-4 people with their arms outstretched to reach around it with their fingertips touching. At between 150-200 years old, they silently graced the side of the hill below the neighboring Chase farm, for generations. When we acquired the land to build the house we often walked out to the old camp through this grove of trees in reverence to their age-old beauty and longevity. Periodically over the years one or two of these trees would succumb to time and the elements and drop their pine needles one last time or topple over into the path that because of their sheer enormity required a great deal of effort to remove. For us, however, this was a labor of love, and we accepted this as the natural course of the elements playing out the normal cycles of birth, life and death.

As we passed often through this grove, we risked picking up deer ticks from the many deer that lived along the river banks. Seldom would they get to actually biting the skin and were promptly removed from our clothing or from our extremities. Just after the land had been purchased, an area along the river was selected and cleared for the house site located just before the pine grove. After work with the chainsaw, the smaller trees were felled and the site was cleared. There was a noticeable increase in the number of ticks found on the work clothes after these sessions. This being 1999, it was more than ever seen before. Eight to ten ticks plucked from the work clothes and sometimes one or two more the next day were found attached to the skin. Of course we were aware of Lyme disease, having experienced it with our daughter Leah some seven years before. This did not thwart my enthusiasm in forging ahead with our plans, however, and the project continued forward.

The house was completed, and we moved in just after year 2000 with all the excitement that comes with enjoying a new home and the fruition of our labor. Our dream house now realized, we accepted with joy the many blessings in seeing it through. Over the next five years we lived happily amongst the trees beside the river with our children, the dogs and the chickens. Yet the underlying feeling of dread and the creeping, pervasive anxiety continued to build during these years and the endless struggle with decisions we had made. Often perplexed why it seemed such an overwhelming struggle, I wondered how to keep it all going. The River Hill band, which after seven years was becoming a thing of the past, now only playing once every couple of months or so and eventually dwindled and fizzled out in 2003. At our last performance at the Barley House in downtown Concord, right across North Main Street from the state capital, I found myself unable to remember the lyrics. The struggle to keep it going became too much, and enjoyment of playing became too burdensome. At the Merrimack Valley School District things were becoming ever more difficult to keep up with, and a breakdown of sorts occurred in the fall of 2004 that sent me home for two months. Sitting by the wood stove stunned for over a month, there was little else that could be done. The multi-family investments were still doing well at the time, but fear of keeping those going also loomed ominously. It seemed for reasons unknown that an inevitable demise was just around the corner, and the race against time and disaster was quickly approaching. The inevitable train wreck was gaining momentum, and there seemed little to do but hold on in desperation for dear life.

With oldest daughter Natalie going to college in Florida and youngest daughter Leah coming up into high school age, though our finances had never been better, my gloomy forecast bloomed like the calm before a storm. The superintendent of schools showed me lists of timber he had sold off his land and recommended finding out whether our property might produce a similar profit from the seven acres of trees along the river. This seemed like a good idea at the time, and we got several loggers to come out and assess the potential for a harvest of the larger trees that had matured. Of course, this included the harvest of the ancient pine grove. We justified this decision by the fact that the grove had reached maturity and in a state of gradual demise, as evidenced by mostly dead limbs up to sparse tops still hosting a bare amount of pine needles. Someday soon these trees would topple in a swift wind anyhow. The thought of profiting on these before they became a burden did much to ease the decision and unburden our conscience. And because we owned both the adjoining pieces of land, the moratorium in the deed for cutting these trees had become moot. We decided to move ahead with the cut.

Dis-employment at Concord Hospital

During the early 1990's while working in the family business "*H.H. Amsden & Sons; Land Surveyors*" there was a deep recession in the nation's economy. With the gloomy economic forecast imminent, one day while standing in the woods by our passive solar home in Epsom, New Hampshire overlooking the hills in the distance across the valley felt as if standing on the edge of an abyss. As pending doom threatened to consume all that we had accomplished, I wrestled with regret for moving back to New Hampshire, and wondered if this was punishment for something that remained unconscious. A feeling of dread became overwhelmingly pervasive, like a thick blanket of dark fog.

While taking classes at Franklin Pierce College, a fellow student, an employee at Concord Hospital, described a position open in the Computer Operations department where she worked and encouraged me to apply for the position. Given the bleak economic circumstances, it was with great relief when the job offer came through, and it was gratefully accepted with new optimism. While at work about a year later, that fateful day when learning of daughter Leah's diagnosis with Lyme will never be forgotten. It was in the basement of the hospital that housed the Computer Operations department, it was mid-morning about 10:00am when the call from the family physician came. He was admitting Leah to the ER immediately for IV treatment, and upon learning this I went could not contain my concern. Overcome with panic and despondency, this was expressed openly in front of co-workers who were shocked, and the look of dismay on their faces reflected the anguish caused by my uncontrolled emotional outburst. Eventually calming down, this was not the last outburst that betrayed inner conflicts at work. There is no room to make excuses. The people who knew me well understood and accepted it, but mere acquaintances and co-workers often seemed repulsed.

"What the hell is wrong with me?"

A frequent mantra, a self-deprecating form of maladjusted behavior began to form as a result. The struggle with this continued throughout the next two jobs in technology. Despite new opportunities to climb out of the hole dug by my own hand, the downward spiral toward inevitable demise betrayed again and again attempts to recreate a new identity. Attitude was hardly coming from the sunny side of the street during those days and compensating to get along with my co-workers and employers would inevitably succumb to a miserable fate beyond any attempts to control it.

"Ralph"

Ralph was our first dog when we migrated back to New Hampshire in the fall of 1988, from Columbia, Maryland. He was a mutt, part German Shepherd, Labrador and Husky, which was a good combination for our growing family of kids, chickens and ducks. As a pup, he was exuberant and willful, and being inexperienced in raising and handling dogs I was sometimes strong handed in my efforts to curb his over-exuberance. Though my methods were not excessively cruel or repressive, there were times when a growing anger would overcome better judgment and would resort to yelling or physical roughness during times of exasperation due to lack of patience. This was not all the time, and there were many occasions of loving kindness and deference to what is, after all, a natural excitability on the part of his doggy nature. We had the joy of adding another dog, a Golden Retriever, Lab, White Shepherd, Husky mix named Alice, to the family, for the two to enjoy each-other's company. Nonetheless, moodiness would sometimes turn into a mild rage directed at the dogs, and the pattern lacked the better sensibilities of patience, tolerance and forbearance.

It is in retrospect, many years later, that I realize this rage was not due so much to the dog's behavior as it was *my* behavior and my reaction to the situation, slowly succumbing to an unknown affliction. But even now, the attempt to deflect the responsibility and project blame upon the Lyme spirochete is no excuse for what occurred. Warning signals easy to ignore or justify in the emerging chaos.

Erich Fromm discusses the topic of cruelty in some detail from his book *The Anatomy of Human Self-Destructiveness:*

> *"The destructive or cruel person has become so because he lacks the conditions for further growth. Under given circumstances he cannot, as it were, do better. His passions are irrational in terms of the possibilities of man, yet they have their rationality in terms of the particular individual and social situation within which a person lives… It needs to be repeated that life-thwarting passions are as much an answer to man's existential needs as life-furthering passions: they both are profoundly human. The former necessarily develop when the realistic conditions for the realization of the latter are absent. Man the destroyer may be called vicious because destructiveness is a vice; but he is human. … In any case, for a man to be stunted in his growth and become vicious is as much a real possibility as to develop fully and to be productive; the one or the other outcome mainly depends on the presence—or absence—of social condi-*

tions conducive to growth. ... It must at the same time be added that in speaking of social circumstances as being responsible for man's development, I do not imply that he is the helpless object of circumstances. Environmental factors (such as neurophysiological) further or hinder the development of certain traits and set the limits within which man acts. Nevertheless, man's reason and will are powerful factors in the process of his development, individually and socially. It is not history that makes man; man creates himself in the process of history."

We are nonetheless responsible and accountable for our actions, reactions or inactions.

From T. Dobzhansky, 1962:

> *"Man knows that he is accountable for his acts: he has acquired the knowledge of good and evil. This is a dreadfully heavy load to carry. No other animal has to withstand anything like it.* **There is tragic discord in the soul of man.** *Among the flaws in human nature, this one is far more serious than the pain of childbirth."*

The LP Compilation Projects with Stellar Voice Productions, Inc.

Prior to coming back to New Hampshire from Maryland in 1988, we spent the previous six years running our company, Stellar Voice Productions, Inc., producing compilation LP records. Those days brought many sublime moments of challenge and victory that fulfilled our wildest dreams. Not only at the time a musician having mastered guitar and synthesizer, our ventures into performing and playing synth techno-pop as the band Stellar Voice had emerged into a higher calling to produce compilation albums during the mid-80's. An exciting time of life, there was a lot going on and many contacts and relationships with other artists and musicians were established. The vinyl LP records were still common during the 1980's and would offer up to 12-14 songs, or more on each record. Depending on the average length of the song, about an hour's worth of playing and listening time was possible.

Daytime work at the NASA Goddard Space Flight Center in Greenbelt, Maryland continued in the real world. Early evening until usually 1:00am or later was spent as a musician and record producer of our small indie-label Empire Records International, producing bands and various musical groups in recording studios in the Washington, DC and Baltimore area. Producing and publishing records that now included bands from all over the country and Canada. Having attained international status was a feather in the cap during those days, as the compilation LPs "*Shades Of The Future*" (1986) was released, "*Dream Sequence*" in (1987), "*In Between The Lines*" (1988), and finally "*Remnants Of A Higher Culture*" in (1990) released on the newest medium known as the CD–compact disc. In the early days of 1990, during the production of "*Remnants*," after reviewing over 900 songs submitted in the mail for consideration for inclusion on the album, there began an increasingly noticeable crushing weight that was difficult to describe other than vaguely some kind of burnout. Pressure from many late nights with Stellar Voice Productions combined with a full-time day job takes its toll even for an otherwise robust 29-year-old.

We shifted responsibilities of the second phase of production to the partner and vice-president of Stellar Voice Productions, and we prepared our escape to New Hampshire in late 1988. We were also to expand the music business geographically to include the Boston and New York areas, as we had several bands published on the LP projects in those locations. And yet, despite the efforts to step back, recuperate and move forward with these life-decisions, the seed of an underlying feeling of a small but persistent desperation had been planted.

New Identity: Dragon-Slayer of the Past

With wisdom comes sorrow.

Recognition of this new role began with resignation from my position as network administrator for Merrimack Valley on July 1, 2006, going back on a promise to *never* leave this job unless terminated by the School Board. This was the first of several promises that could not be kept. Earlier while visiting the White Mountains with my faithful Newfoundland, we hiked up to Greeley Pond to contemplate this decision. There seemed no alternative to this agonizing decision. A creeping form of incompetence had mysteriously arisen, seemingly from nowhere and taken over. My identity, who I thought I was, no longer existed, and the man I had become was like an *empty shell*. Walking the paths in desperation along the Blackwater River during those last days brought on a suffocating feeling of not having enough air and a crushing weight on the chest. An escape plan had become a matter of *survival*.

Next came a complete role-reversal, taking a job as caretaker of a bamboo farm in Florida. The transition to Florida began, and tenants were found to occupy the home of our dreams, which we were leaving behind. Thus began a "new life" in a desperate last-ditch attempt to recreate myself. In complete contrast to the prior twenty-five years, it was a huge relief from the crushing load now left behind.

Positive for advanced, late-stage Lyme disease.
"Old" Lyme.

Never will be forgotten that moment of truth. Such a combination and tangle of emotions: relief, anguish, despair, hope, confusion, exasperation, anger, disbelief. Hope emerged briefly for an instant, that there might be a way out of this nightmare. Immediately, plans were made to return to New Hampshire and begin treatment. The antiques were sold at auction and meager possessions packed in a U-Haul truck. Creeping slowly north for the next three days through inclement icy weather and treacherous roads, it was a tenuous trip, and the pain, anxiety and fatigue were at their peak. As the role of dragon-slayer of my own creations came to a close, it was my last major undertaking for the next seven years.

As the Silent Epidemic Continues

"…And I set my mind to seek and explore by wisdom concerning all that has been done under heaven. It is a grievous task which God has given to the sons of men to be afflicted with. I have seen all the works which have been done under the sun, and behold, all is vanity and striving after wind. What is crooked cannot be straightened and what is lacking cannot be counted…"
—Ecclesiastes

A stunning silence beckons the monster across nearly every threshold, impacting every citizen either personally or indirectly. The costs to individuals and society are beyond measure, the least of which is financial. The toll measured in misery and missed opportunity is colossal. The effect on future generations, devastating.

Truth, as understood in the divine sphere, is immutable, eternal, and never-changing. It stands as the beacon of everlasting life, in sharp contradistinction to the perpetual cycles of birth-life-death that characterizes the physical world. Despite our vain attempts through science, much as we try to control the external forces of nature we are more often misled by our senses than saved by them. In our frantic and arrogant attempts to impose our will on the world, karmic debt is incurred upon ourselves and others, the consequences of which is suffering.

Could this be the actual source of our conflict, not just of the current Lyme dilemma, but for all similar dilemmas, past, present and future? This calls for scrutiny, as the possible origin and history of the human species in war, pestilence, poverty and famine. These four horseman of the Apocalypse are ever-present to ensure and restore the balance and harmony between Nature and the Divine, to atone for actions and reactions between ignorance and understanding, denial and compassion. Perhaps it is ours to alter this formula and throw universal harmony out of balance but also to create that opportunity to change ourselves from within as a consequence.

Within, we restore the balance and thereby reflect in the world our deepest desires for peace, harmony, justice, health—in other words, we hold within ourselves the formula of our own *well-being*. We hold within ourselves this power. It is not found "out there" as we have been lead to believe.

Could this be the key to our understanding not only Lyme specifically, but human suffering in general?

As with all such trials and tribulations, we continue to suffer at the invisible hand of something seemingly just beyond human comprehension. Our belief in what we understand as reality is not always as they appear, and this is for good reason. Extremely difficult to comprehend and understand, this is even more difficult to accept. Ignoring the calls from our own soul, the small voice within, the voice of conscience for a new dialogue about life denies the gifts of the divine, and has its consequences:

Carl Jung continues:

> *"Human thought cannot conceive any system or final truth that could give the patient what he needs in order to live: that is faith, hope, love and insight. These four greatest achievements of human effort are so many gifts of grace, which are neither to be taught nor learned, neither given [by us] nor taken, neither withheld or earned, since they come through experience, which is something given, and therefore beyond the reach of human ca-*

price. Experiences cannot be made. They can only be accepted."

Alan Watts suggests in his book "*Behold the Spirit*" that the mystical union of the suffering spirit with the divine soul be the primary act, or purpose, to achieve meaning in life after being separated from itself. That suffering has its place in the human experience; that our efforts, deliberately or otherwise, persist as human suffering when we fail to recognize well-being as a natural condition of our existence:

> *".... It is a fruit of union that men should desire to heal the sick and to prolong life and health. It is a fruit of union that they should study the secrets of nature and develop sciences and still to this end. But when these goals are pursued for their own sake, when their original impulse and their final end are forgotten and untaught, the power of healing becomes a power of destruction. It is a fruit of union that men should study agriculture and engineering to feed the hungry and clothe the naked, but when the object of production becomes "living for back and belly" - the moral impulse has failed in its object and become positively immoral...."*

According to Fromm, our culture of malignant narcissism and self-destruction reveals an afflicted and unrestrained ego, based upon the cultural characteristics of sadism (the impulse to force and control the will of others), masochism (the tendency to submit to the doctrine of an external authority over the individual), and necrophilia (the "death instinct" discovered by Freud.) Not inherent in man's instinctive nature, but *learned* and nurtured through cultural and environmental conditions we call "civilization," we ourselves are responsible for what Alan Watts describes as reactionary phenomena in the struggle against or resistance to the divine will:

> *"Especially is this true in regards to suffering, for suffering is transformed and its meaning realized only when the sufferer affirms it as the divine will. To struggle against inevitable pain is only to intensify grief and when the moment brings pain the praise of God consists in entering into its very heart, cooperate with it, and telling it to be as painful as it takes. At first thought this seems madness itself to the sufferer, but the total acceptance and affirmation of pain is the essence...In these circumstances what we are to accept is not so much the pain itself as our own reaction to it, to fight and to flee. When this is done we discover*

invariably that God permits us to suffer in order to 'debunk' our egoism, and that this is mercy itself because it opens our eyes to his splendor and love, giving it an infinite joy in return for a finite pain. There is no proof of this truth but experiment."

Could this "total acceptance and affirmation of pain" be the reluctance of some to become well again? In my case, as with many Lyme sufferers with no capability to move or do anything, this is difficult to accept. Facing this possibility reflected in the mirror of experience takes supreme effort to first even consider, and even more to comprehend, understand and finally, accept. Objective critical analysis and willingness to accept those conclusions requires a rare courage. Many months of virtual paralysis from pain, anxiety, depression and profound fatigue offered little choice but to accept this condition and retreat within. It was *there* and then that my recovery truly began. Regrouping in new surroundings and acceptance of my condition of suffering prepared me for a long, long wait. It was *there* that patience, forbearance, tolerance, humility, acceptance, gratitude and faith came. Faith in something greater than the trappings and illusions of the material world emerged. It was *there* that a new set of values began to surface in consciousness. This is what is described in the transmutation of metals in alchemy; the ascension of the soul in Gnostic literature; the Crucifixion and Resurrection and being "reborn" in Christian theology; the state of "transmigration of the soul" in eastern theology; the heavenly city of the 18th century philosophers; the new Jerusalem of the Pentecost.

A new message from the small voice within said:

"The answers we so desperately seek in the external world are found within."

Further reflected in the Erich Fromm's book "*The Anatomy of Human Self-destructiveness*" published in 1973, Fromm makes an important distinction between Freud's "death instinct" as inherent in human instinct opposed to Fromm's theory that *learned tendencies* of sadism, masochism and necrophilia occur as a result of cultural and environmental values. His thorough analysis and critique of these human tendencies and the subsequent differentiation of these sources of suffering as *learned tendencies* belong to the environmental social-conditions of civilization, and *do not exist* in human instincts of self-preservation and self-defense. This is an important distinction and refutation of the Freudian concept of evil instincts as inherent in man's nature and will take decades if not centuries to undo. Nonetheless, this is an important discovery for a new understanding of our position and role in creation, its meaning and our purpose.

Advancement of human knowledge in physical and social sciences continue to challenge the status quo of dogma and doctrine, comprising the values and principles of human society. That we are primarily the cause of our own conditions challenges what we have been taught to believe, generation after generation. To consider alternatives, to look at ourselves introspectively with a critical eye and with inner contemplation, we must seek the *enemy within*.

The Enemy Within

> *"I have seen all the works that are done under the sun; and, behold, all is vanity and vexation of spirit."*
> *—Ecclesiastes 1:14*

Superstition continues to play a primary role in social values rooted in the character of modern urban society. These root causes are typical of the ignorance and denial mirrored in the underlying problem of Lyme disease. We see this as symptomatic of manifestations of the spirit, reflected in the individual character of modern man, both a creature of instinct and environment. Mankind nonetheless displays character traits that originate from the spirit, and these are reflected in our social institutions; in economics, politics, education, medicine and religion. From the earliest development of human civilization, we see the shocking increase of violence and destruction against our own kind. It reveals the anemic presence of a sickly collective human spirit, acquiescent to the onslaughts of our own devices in technology and science. This perpetual cycle of self-destruction is increasing in its severity and depravity, revealing the parasitic nature of predatory forces that feed on misery and suffering of our own making. Carl Jung speaks of this duality of human nature in the following words:

> *"But if we can reconcile ourselves with the mysterious truth that spirit is the living body seen from within, and the body the outer manifestation of the spirit – the two really one – then we can understand why it is that the attempt to transcend the present level of consciousness must give its due to the body. We shall*

also see that belief in the body cannot tolerate an outlook that denies the body in the name of the spirit. These claims of physical and psychic life are so pressing compared to similar claims in the past, that we are tempted to see in this a sign of decadence. Yet it may also signify a rejuvenation, for as Holderlin says: "Danger itself fosters the rescuing power."

What we actually see is that the Western world strikes up a still more rapid tempo – the American tempo – the very opposite of quietism and resigned aloofness. An enormous tension arises between the opposite poles of outer and inner life, between the objective and subjective reality."

We see this same trend also in politics. As it has been said in politics, *power corrupts, and absolute power corrupts absolutely.*

We also see the same pattern persists in the advancement and progress of the physical sciences. Our spiritual nature substituted for devotion to materialism and excessive consumerism is dragged down again and again by the anchor of power and politics. Human culture today worships and rewards the values of competition, aggression, and divisiveness over cooperation, collaboration and unity. Spiritual values such as compassion, charity and forgiveness are marginalized, denigrated, even ridiculed. The insidious degeneration of human society preaches the virtues of advances in science and civilization, while unseen parasitic and predatory forces continue to profit on human misery and suffering. Jung summarizes:

"The science of medicine has avoided all contact with strictly psychic problems."

There is no exception to this reality to be found in modern medicine. Here, too, the values of egoism accumulate material wealth and power at the expense of well-being. There is no "health-care" currently in modern society. At best there is a "sick-care" where symptoms are relieved while protecting and nurturing the origin of disease. This is not difficult to understand. There is no money to be made from otherwise healthy individuals in health-care. Well-being is a loser on the stock market. Our age is marked by the Golden Egg of the sick goose, where profit is idolized and worshiped over well-being.

While the 20th century remains forever marred by this shameful affair, it cannot continue to merely treat symptoms while ignoring root causes. Real change poses a threat to its dominance in the pharmaceutical industries and treatment facilities. Fearing reprisal should we expose it for what it is—a deception of the worst possible kind—here again we encounter the *"lie too big to admit."*

To suddenly confront denial would implicate our own part in this clever self-deception. Our own gullibility implicates ourselves as the origin of our own suffering. How could we possibly admit this to ourselves?

The Dilemma of Modern Medicine

"First do no harm." —the Hippocratic Oath

Tainted by money and unimpeded accumulation of power and wealth, we see this not only in Lyme, but in the cancer and chronic disease industries. Demanding compliance with policies that are intended to undermine genuine health and well-being, we also see this in the food industry, modern agriculture methods, education and particularly in government. Focusing on treating symptoms, while systemically denying the cure, is in effect making a killing for those invested in treatment over cure.

The modern myth of "health-care" is a long-way from being realized as a transformative reality. Despite over 300-years of scientific advancement, the reality of our spiritual reality continues to be largely ignored by mainstream science. This is starting to change. Yet, these discoveries and advances have a tendency to serve the wrong master. In many ways controlled by monetary interests, these motivations benefit the few at the expense of the many. Testimonies to greed and vanity, modern science in medicine remain underscored by a lack of vision. Values and principles that should benefit all, and not just the interests of the few, are influenced and co-opted by special interests—a game that has been well played successfully over and over. But, we are fooling no one but ourselves. Denial of these facts continues only to serve the interests of the few; refusal to accept these truths only harms those who deny them.

Though evidence is slow to be revealed, we should know from past experience that it has become necessary to influence our own destiny either passively as victims of fate or by actively *choosing* a destiny that reflects a higher purpose to truly live in a light of consciousness that transcends the false-self ego. Until recognized and accepted, the *status quo* will continue to dominate the individual mind with distraction, temptation, bribery, and extortion. How much longer can we afford to fool ourselves? We obfuscate this reality in our everyday life, choosing safety and comfort while permitting our subconscious to be manipulated and exploited. Remaining hidden from sight, we continue to define ourselves with false justifications of necessity and self-preservation. By this clever self-deception we continue to justify and excuse desire for money, power and control. Permitted to reside in the sub-conscious through submission, these unconscious acts, when faced directly and intentionally, are brought into the light of pure consciousness. This is the method by which we transform ourselves, and thereby transform the world we live in.

This recognition and acknowledgement arrives with new responsibilities. Deep within ourselves, and ultimately towards mankind itself, in light of our false-beliefs and egocentric values we currently embrace, we begin to see things in a different way. Negative character traits we stubbornly cling to are exposed from within, and the rug is pulled out from under us. The shaky pillars of illusion buckle and fall in a new understanding of our condition. To know this intuitively on a transcendental level is to understand the divine principle of creation and evolution of the spirit, and a new understanding of why we are here. What gives meaning and purpose to a rational existence in a world of constant change and distraction is our understanding of this.

We have the power to create the conditions of the world we exist in through our ideas of what the world would be.

Our thoughts originate from ideas. The thoughts by our imagination create the ideas we enshroud ourselves in every day. Where beliefs no longer serve our interests today as individual spiritual beings, it requires us to examine them critically and exercise judgment. At this point we determine our direction—toward self-deception and the consequences of depravity and suffering or recognition of our birthright toward compassion and understanding.

The enemy within that guards our modern tendency toward egoism is two headed. One head is called Ignorance, the other, Denial. They are both self-serving and reinforce each other. This is a creature of and by our own hands and continues to thrive as we cultivate and nurture it. Sacrificed on the altar of science, faith known intuitively is measured by these acts.

But science that stands on that which cannot be measured does not currently exist, and thereby continues to reject the deeper truths of ourselves. Comfortably concealed behind its robe of ignorance and denial, this Goliath lurks invisibly in the collective unconscious where it remains nurtured unwittingly by us, just below the surface of our awakened consciousness. Meanwhile, the inherent tendency to believe what we are told in blind trust is repeated over and over. Promising that domination of nature is *absolutely necessary* for survival becomes the basis of our self-destruction, and the wheel of self-deception continues in a self-fulfilling cycle.

And yet, it is *precisely these* experiences that have been most useful and possess the most value in understanding our purpose, that give meaning to our lives. It is from this dimension of reality that the struggle for consciousness arises. Transforming ourselves, and society accordingly, occurs by raising awareness by degree of our human consciousness *first within ourselves*. To re-create life based upon a new paradigm of vastly different principles and values, we contemplate inwardly a new dialogue from the one we have been taught since birth. The current emphasis and insistence upon the materialistic dialectic of nature has become the *source* of our physical (and spiritual) suffering. Constant emphasis and reinforcement of negative evolutionary values expressed by this two-headed Goliath characterizes our current version of reality. To overcome this and create a new reality requires re-evaluation of our individual goals and values in understanding how these contribute to society at large and beginning a new narrative that expresses these.

This new narrative as relates to Lyme suggests that somehow the financial incentive to *treat* illness and the idea that we must battle against disease instead of battling for a *cure* must be removed or transformed. The medical community itself and the vast network of health-care systems of insurance and government agencies—entities purported to be in the best interest of the people—are in fact promoted by rampant self-interest. To create a system of actual health-care, a new direction and reorientation toward *well-being* must occur. The current emphasis on intentional suffering, by focusing exclusively on treatment of symptoms for financial gain, must be discontinued.

Too much money is being made keeping people sick.

To break the current pattern and emerge from this paradigm of financial predation requires the will to act. The rise in many immunodeficient diseases we are experiencing are a direct result of this current health-care debacle.

While assessing the current health-care system crisis, though highly critical of its shortcomings, it is important also to recognize dedicated individuals who are truly seeking positive change in research and development of new cures and alternative treatments. Creating options to corporate-controlled care is certainly revolutionary considering the many industries and institutions that profit by its contrary. As with all things that seem "tainted by money," money in and of itself is only incidental to the problem, it is how money is used that ultimately determines the outcome.

Again, we see here the source of illness as an affliction of the spiritual nature of mankind. Its source resides in the principles and values we embrace and the consequences therein, whether influenced by the two-headed Goliath or by the spiritual soul which connects us all. *Ultimately we are the source of the affliction that our spirit suffers.* Our actions determined by the will are a direct reflection of the principles and values we embrace within ourselves. As individuals that comprise our greater human society, to consider the source of our principles and values, what do we value? We tend to worship the ideals of materialism in modern society, mostly advanced by the glamour and material rewards of modern science.

> *Could this be key to comprehending and understanding the underlying source of our self-deception, our learned tendencies of self-destruction and intentional suffering?*

Subject to an external world that influences and directly impacts our daily lives, it is simply reflecting values that we embrace from either the ego or the spirit. It is ultimately our choice.

PART 7

The Secret Gift of Lyme

"Vanity of vanities, all is vanity."
—Ludwig Wittgenstein

Extremely counter-intuitive at first, enduring misery and suffering is our greatest gift.

Returning to Florida after twenty-four months of treatment took an act of will that seemed at first impossible. Still mostly paralyzed and bed-ridden, the relentless and excruciating Herx effects from treatment were completely debilitating. About 95% disabled, prevailing with Social Security Disability afforded the opportunity to reinvent life again and escape the dreaded cold of New England. Getting around was more like a 90-year-old man with AIDS than a fifty-one-year-old just coming out of the prime of life. Crippled and bent over, with the help of a cane, walks around the neighborhood were endured but with little enjoyment. Yet, there was deep inside a determination to move forward with life, such as it was, and begin to free myself from the past.

Finding a competent Lyme-literate doctor in Florida was a miracle in and of itself. Joining a Lyme support group in Naples produced a tip for an infectious disease doctor in Lakeland, about 1.5 hours from Inverness, where I now lived. The first appointment was made after assurance that this doctor was experienced in Lyme and claimed to have successfully treated over 500 patients with Borrelia. He was in his seventies, experienced and unafraid of aggressively tackling the problem head-on. He praised my first doctor for setting me on the right path. Doxycycline was added to the protocol, 200mg. twice per day, and Amytriptline for the dreaded dysautonia that plagued every waking moment. Clonazepam and Adderall were continued, as was Prozac for depression, and the Lyrica for pain established some balance to the daily waves of dread, anxiety and pain that threatened to engulf everything without them. Arms, elbows, forearms, wrists, knuckles felt as though pounded by a rubber mallet. Excruciating pain in the nerves, as though being constantly electrocuted. The constant jolts, brain zaps, min-convulsions and temporary seizures that began as a child over forty years before now had me completely and utterly incompetent. A speech impediment similar to Tourette-syndrome silenced most conversation, and life chained to the couch watching TV became the only thing left to do.

This new infectious disease doctor claimed a 90-95% chance of a full recovery, a *cure*, even in my advanced condition. I replied that I hadn't heard the "c" word very much in my experience so far and felt encouraged by his confidence and optimism. New hope appeared on the horizon as I implored "how much longer?" His honesty was refreshing. Though it was now just over two years into treatment, he predicted months—possibly many more months—years—to reach the finish line. He admonished that it took a long time to get into this condition, and it was going to take a lot of time to get out of it.

Meanwhile, the treatment continued under his close supervision, and each month returning to his office became every three months. It was still difficult most of the time, if not impossible, to tell whether the tide was coming in or going out. As time passed, I noticed an ever so slight improvement in certain things; a returning of the ability to think, to feel, to observe… Endurance returned almost imperceptibly at first, as did the ability to reason and the will. I began re-finishing antiques again and opened a spot at Traditions, a large antique outlet located in Wildwood, to sell them. Over the next year, the proceeds were used to purchase a piece of land in Inverness at auction. I never thought I would ever own property again.

This was encouraging, indeed. But, the constant agony endured went on for nearly another two years. At forty-four months of steady, uninterrupted treatment, my doctor announced he was retiring in September of 2012. During the summer there was some debate over whether the finish line had been crossed, and he prescribed a strong antibiotic called Flagyl to eradicate the cystic form of the disease. It affected my sinuses and lungs in a way not previously experienced. The sensation one has emerging from a chlorinated swimming pool comes to mind. The brain-stem headaches and crushing fatigue that destabilized much of my overall condition were beginning to fade, and the feeling in the arms of being constantly tortured by electrocution was also noticeably less. Meanwhile, a date at "Crackers" restaurant in Crystal River turned out to introduce me to my new life-partner Pam, and things seemed to really be turning around.

The Lyme debacle is but a symptom of a much larger issue. It is symptomatic of an affliction of the human spirit that permeates our collective consciousness, that *we* are the source of. "*Vanity, vanity, vanity…. all is vanity.*" How often we have heard the phrase but refuse to understand it. Erroneous confidence in *our false pride*, our limited and deceptive senses and the blind acceptance of principles and values that our existence owes only to the physical world is what obscures the ultimate truth about ourselves. Sustained reliance of our egocentric nature is *designed* to obscure the omnipresence and eternal reality about our true being. All around us and within us the presence of this reality exists, unrecognized and unaccepted. We are spiritual beings born of compassion and love.

What the eyes alone see is not what the soul desires. Our earthly physical existence is primarily occupied with and dominated by concerns, rather than cultivating the needs of the spirit. We tend to cherish our earthly works, rather than the virtues of selflessness, charity, generosity and compassion. The great wheel of karma and reincarnation adjusts all such imbalances. How it does this? Through the Four Horsemen of the Apocalypse:

War, poverty, disease and famine.

By these four horsemen driving the forces of Karma, we derive our greatest gifts. The answers to our dilemma would not exist without them. It is by way of struggle and the challenges that overcome resistance and interference that we rise to the occasion of our own soul's ascension back to the divine. The mystic's journey is *everyone's* journey. It is the purpose of our existence, our reason for being born into this world, and the guiding light that leads us back from whence we came. The lessons obtained while living in the world of generated existences furnishes our soul with the opportunity to learn through experience our true selves, our true nature, and the power and the glory that resides within every person. The great gifts that have been bestowed upon us are available to all, whether we are in a position to accept them or not is what makes all the difference. The cycles of life ensure that all will eventually receive them, whether in this life, the next, or those that follow. We need not fear, as joy and suffering are but two sides of the same coin. And once we rise again, step forward and embrace our true heritage, we accept what is ours to begin with, through recognition, acceptance and *gratitude*.

The "secret gifts of Lyme" from this journey comprise too many to mention here. These need not be limited to the consequences of Lyme disease, but disease in general and all that challenge the soul's life in the return home. These lamps lit by experience of the spiritual illuminate the path to the kingdom within, the Eden we were cast out of, the Kingdom of Heaven that resides within every human being. We are Divine.

My journey is testament to this, as I am its living witness.

Cure Unknown, or Cure Denied?

The essence of human nature is often contrary to what appears in the phenomenal world, as witnessed by history and the ever-changing present. In the beginning, the soul's journey home is often characterized by an occurrence or event of a revelatory nature. No matter how well managed our planned lives go, we all experience what at first appears as a principle of random discord, where nature seems to generate accidents or events that randomly influence our direction. These appear to be self-inflicted at times yet can also appear as external events. These events form the basis for the lessons presented to us as opportunities for learning and understanding. It is our divine nature that is revealed in these lessons—a recognition and acceptance of that which has been bestowed upon us. It is the indwelling eternal presence that resides in each one of us that guides our soul's journey. To surmount the challenges presented to us evolves our consciousness from a state of slumber to greater awareness. The evolution of mankind *is* the evolution of soul-consciousness. The cure is known, but denied.

Humility—"Vanity (Pride) Goest Before A Fall"

"Pride goeth before destruction, and a haughty spirit before a fall."
—Proverbs 16:18

Nothing is more humbling than a disease that removes one from all they have attained and accomplished. To make this point, many times during our brief lives we encounter accomplishments and victories, providing a false sense of omnipotence. In that end, it makes us foolish. Sacrifice is by intent, yet the humbleness earned by unintentional loss ever reminds us of our fragile condition and position in the shadow world of appearances.

Most all of us initially take a lot of interest in how we appear to others, a cloak of self-deception we offer to others for appearances sake. We tend to pick out attractive people to admire, and perhaps only later we learn that looks are not as important as the wisdom, health, and vocation of the inner person—the *real* person. In our world of contrast, we often subject ourselves to this form of vanity, not just in appearances but in our efforts. The apparition of self-importance creates itself as a warm and inviting abode for the ego's delusional nature and continues its illusion of itself. To the point where we deceive ourselves, we are set up for a lesson in humility. The aforementioned Four Horsemen ensure this, and Karma is ultimately successful in restoring balance in our true nature. Our selfish pride, the vanity of our arrogance, is the primary source of ill-health and disease. They prepare the ground for vice and sow the seed of the inevitable weeds and vines that will overtake us. To prepare fertile ground for virtue to take root, we become better gardeners of the garden within. To improve the Garden, first improve the Gardener.

The Imperative of Patience

As neuro-borreliosis manifests in multiple forms of debilitation, impatience can become our own worst enemy. With spirochetes flourishing in the nervous system, it is small wonder it has this effect on the brain and the personality. *Anxiety and depression* are expressed differently but often share the root of unbalanced but justified concern for ourselves. Overly concerned with how our image appears to others, concealing our true identity of inner suffering and weakness becomes increasingly imperative. Lessons of tolerance and forbearance result from this lack of patience. We become "patients" to our doctors and our caretakers when these lessons are ignored. Intolerance due to lack of respect for ourselves and others is born of denial, a deliberate ignorance of others' place and position in the soul-ascension. Not everyone is at the same level of spiritual high ground. Recognizing and understanding this, first about ourselves then others, leads to the still waters of self-reflection and acceptance of others' concerns as our own.

Having Lyme exacerbates these symptoms to an extreme. Yet, through the lessons of humility and patience we are provided the opportunity to overcome these weaknesses in our own soul. If we listen carefully and learn to "see" with the eyes of our spirit, we become aware of these lessons and embrace them with gratitude, in spite of the physical suffering incurred. It is not easy to overcome long-term habits, and sometimes requires extreme measures to not only face them, but transform ourselves in the process to *overcome* them. The method can seem harsh, and of necessity it is, but offers the opportunity of transmutation that would otherwise remain impossible. Patience is a learned behavior. Recovering from a long and debilitating illness renders the opportunity for great learning of the lessons of patience. But, it us up to us to recognize this and not let it pass us by.

The Flowers of Charity and Generosity

From the mud and the muck arises the flower, and so it is with the flowers of charity and generosity. Blossoming forth from the tendencies of "what is mine is mine" and the worn-out welcome of survival of the fittest, those who have run the gauntlet of loss have a new appreciation for what is. A propensity to share what is no longer theirs emerges as lessons for those who have attained and acquired much. It seems natural at first that hard work earns what is ours. The human tendency to protect what is "rightly" ours comes from the material world of *things* and is reinforced by civil law, private property rights and fueled by the notion of *necessity*. But how do we know what is really necessary until we go without? The cult of personality so predominant during our modern age provides a disturbed foundation prone to decay and disease. The more the false-self ego is invested in its shaky confidence, the harder the fall when the rug is pulled out from under. *Thus, it is in the ground furrowed by the plow of humility that the seeds of charity and generosity are planted and born.*

The illusions of wealth and power we use to idolize and justify our arrogance and self-importance underscore our efforts to protect the false-self ego. When the false identity is exposed, understanding that true wealth is found in our service to others who have suffered greater misfortunes than ours gradually emerges. By our great works or our suffering, the karmic debts are paid, and the great balance of nature is continuously restored. We either become part of the healing process or recipients of it. The harvest is more often the unseen works of our compassion than the work of our hands, yet both are required.

Giving as a selfless act of compassion and empathy nurtures not only those who are influenced by it but our own soul as well. We who have been robbed of our material possessions have the opportunity to understand this in a new light. When all we have worked for in the material world and have invested our time in comes to naught, what is *really* important suddenly emerges with new clarity. For those who experience this, it is a blessing, not a curse. Our biggest and most challenging lesson often comes of tragedy and loss; such as experienced by loss of health.

As the saying goes in the song "Scarlet Begonias" by the Grateful Dead:

"Once in a while you get shown the light,
in the strangest places if you look at it right."

No Shame: Our Purpose—Forgiveness and Redemption

It becomes so easy to overlook what is really important when things seem to be going well. The myriad of distractions and forces that influence our behavior on a daily basis keep us focused on the trivial and meaningless and away from the more important issues of our lives. Created dependencies from advances in science and technology keep our nose pointed into the winds of change as time marches on with or without us in the other direction. Ever fearful those winds may change unfavorably, we withdraw into ourselves while maintaining our sight outwards, as protection from fear of that change. We build a false wall around ourselves, concealed behind a wall of shame, in disgrace for the fear and denial we put into nurturing our false-self ego. The malignant narcissism so characteristic of our current modern age is nurtured by us. The amount of wasted energy poured into this futile effort is enormous.

That there be more to this hardly occurs to us during our daily struggles but comes to us in the early hours of the morning, as when awakened by a nightmare. Threats of potential loss of what we have built up through our toil and hard work creep in from the back of the mind where we spend so much time and energy keeping it buried. When others pose threats to our security, we tend to fearfully lash out in retaliation or revenge, justified as self-defense or justice deserved. These are common reactions to protection of our false-security, reinforced by civil law and justified by social norms. Yet, it is only by our recognition of this, and by heroic acts of forgiveness, tolerance and temperance, that we are truly set free. The more acrimony and antipathy we cement into the walls of protection we surround ourselves with, the more the strength of that wall diminishes. When tragedy suddenly strikes, and loss or health are diminished, these new elements begin to erode our walls of protection. Soon the light starts to shine through the chinks of the wall and our own armor begins to rust and corrode. We no longer see our neighbors as a threat but as souls like ourselves with their own struggles and challenges in this life. A new spirit is born within the personality, and a common ground is now recognized between ourselves and others.

Having newly observed that we all share this space and time we call life, a fresh impulse to make amends for wrongs committed against others becomes predominant. Forgiving others' acts of fear and transgressions against us generates a new understanding when we no longer shore up those walls of protection. Reaching out to those that have done a disservice to us not only frees our enemies but liberates our own soul in the process. Selfless acts of compassion now include forgiveness of others, and in the process of setting them free we also do for ourselves. Our contributions to the salvation of those who have wronged us become the basis of our own redemption. To recognize this becomes our purpose in this life.

The hard lessons from the journey, if recognized,
acknowledged and accepted, are the very keys to our
kingdom of paradise. We possess them within.

Acts of Atonement and Liberation of the Spirit

The process of forgiveness changes us from within and becomes part of our daily life. Sometimes when we have suffered loss of all we thought we had—health, friends and possessions, and particularly our identity—the act of forgiving ourselves, as well as others, occurs spontaneously. Acknowledging and accepting others' intentions turned against us goes both ways. In forgiving ourselves for acts committed *against* others we resurrect within ourselves a new life based upon compassion *for* others. These acts of forgiveness often take the form of atonement, a spontaneous form of compassion to make amends for wrongs committed against others. We find within ourselves a new life forming that extends towards others we have wronged, and in so doing nurture each other and ourselves in the process.

Acts of atonement as expression of compassion serves to liberate both the *liberator* and the *liberatee*. When we act with kindness towards one another we give ourselves the opportunity to make right transgressions made and received and present the opportunity to be forgiven for them on both sides. This is the beauty of atonement. It is both an *at-one* with and the setting anew of *a-tone* within others and ourselves. It is adopting a higher energy, a *tone*, that vibrates at a higher frequency, felt by both the *a-toner* and the *a-tonee*. We begin to sing a new tune that resonates in harmony with our universe, and the forces we were once hardened to struggle against soften. We also begin to see changes in the world we thought would never happen. More often about direction than substance, we begin to see a new world emerge from within and enfold in beauty.

These changes frequently do not occur when we have been made comfortable in our surroundings, obscured behind the wall we have built for ourselves. When we are stripped of these, we have a new opportunity to see what exists beyond them—a world that places value on real common ground between ourselves and others. The former illusion of separateness between ourselves and others begins to dissolve, as a clouded veil of mist disperses in the morning light of the rising sun. In a new light, we see what was formerly missing in our lives, the real connection to others and to life itself. Our true human nature is obscured by the veil of illusion that emphasizes the dog-eat-dog world we have been taught to believe.

Yet, because such illusions exist, we are given the lamp of atonement.

The trials and tribulations of our earthly existence, be it illusions of comfort and protection or loss of health by disease, all lead eventually to the same the conclusion: we are not alone in this universe. These are the lessons—our gifts of the soul's journey to liberate the human-spirit.

The Secret Gift: Compassion and Gratitude

Were it not for misfortune, there would be no solace in compassion and gratitude. The lessons in life are the training ground for the soul's ascension, in this life as well as the next. We often fall short of recognizing these hardships as challenges that provide our greatest gifts. The opportunities to gain the pearls of wisdom that transform ourselves from within occur because of these tragedies and misfortunes. When the seed of transformation planted within our soul is nurtured by acts of compassion, we offer gratitude to all that we come in contact with. As part of the transformation process, our lives become an expression of gratitude itself. Living in compassion and gratitude becomes a gift in and of itself. These two acts nurture each other in an endless expansion of love and kindness, towards ourselves and others, and is reflected in the universe at large.

Gradually we come to realize that our acts determine the consequences of the so-called "outside" world, reflected back upon us. These are the karmic laws of nature that have been by deliberately left out of our education textbooks. There are non-human forces hard at work to make sure we do not have the opportunity to understand these things. This is so for very good reason. Jealousy and envy so prevalent in the ordinary consciousness of the daily world provide those opportunities to overcome *ignorance and denial*. They appear as misfortunes and tragedies of an accidental nature but are based upon our acts of will and designed to plant the impulse to seek something more. They are the cause of our greatest gifts. This is the great secret behind not just Lyme disease, but behind *human suffering in general.* It is by the lessons of misfortune that we find our higher path to redemption. That we are all creatures of the divine essence is the crowning glory of recognition. We are *all* on the same path. Compassion and gratitude become habituated in the soul through practice. Practice means changing our thinking, developing intuition, and nurturing inspiration. It is about the impulse to become something better.

Three Keys to the Kingdom: Recognition, Acknowledgement and Acceptance

The illusion of separateness, eventually acknowledged by all, will be recognized for what it is: an illusion. This is inevitable if we first recognize, acknowledge, and finally, accept it fully. Understand that returning to this existence in the physical world in numerous other lives is essential. All are not on the same level of ascension of the spiritual path in this life, but we are not doomed in perpetuity as a result of it. This can be most difficult to recognize, acknowledge and accept. We have been taught since birth the grand illusion that we exist but once in the physical world, and through fear we are manipulated, exploited and controlled to the degree that we have been taught to believe only what others have chosen for us to believe. We do not learn the universal truth regarding the power of our own free will in school, in church, or from our social institutions, as those are designed to *prevent* the understanding of this. It is essential that those institutions pose as beneficial to us, in fact, they will expend any and all means to ensure that you understand how *absolutely essential* it is to protect and defend the status quo. In fact, it is *required by law,* at all costs—even if it costs everything. But, we can begin to see from this narrative why this is so.

It is so for good reason, though typically we do not recognize it as such because we have been taught not to recognize it this way. This is a great lesson for us to learn. *We* actually possess the power to change the world as we know it. Recall that when one wishes to improve the Garden, one must begin with the Gardener. By tending the Garden Within, the Observer is changed, and thereby what the Observer/Gardener observes has changed. This change is reflected in our world, our world of ordinary everyday consciousness—what we typically refer to as "reality." What we typically refer to as "reality" actually is merely the *reflection* of what is real, a mirror image of what *is*. This is us. Each one of us. It is at first a difficult concept to comprehend, but with inner contemplation the idea reveals itself gradually.

These forces represent reflection from within,
the consequences of our thoughts and actions
that result from their images projected back upon us
from the reflected mirror of 'reality'.

Were even an insignificant portion of humanity to recognize and understand this, much misery and suffering in the world, particularity in the forms of violence, war and poverty, would cease immediately. The level of suffering endured currently would decrease significantly as recognition increased in proportion. But until recognition, acknowledgement and acceptance become a reality, we will continue the path in the wrong direction—ignorance, self-denial, the path for self-destruction.

Meanwhile, as we gradually recognize our own worst enemy in us, we continue to sacrifice *everything* for it. Our freedom, our individual sovereignty, our health, our wealth, even our lives are sacrificed out of our own birth rights as a citizen of this earth? Yet, these exist for a reason.

They are to prod us onto the path of redemption through acts of forgiveness, atonement and compassion. These, in turn, lead to the recognition, acknowledgment and acceptance of what *is*. The gifts of the universe are bestowed freely and equally upon all. These two sets of realities go hand in hand. One shakes the other. The circle is complete. Ignorance and denial, the source of our own suffering, is resolved in recognition, acknowledgement and acceptance of what *is*. And by this we contemplate what will be.

The Evolution of Consciousness and Transformation of the Self

Intentionally, we create and sustain a quality of life worth living or unknowingly create one unworthy of us. We all carry within us the potential for unconscious self-destruction of ourselves and others, but also the potential for conscious self-awareness of the soul and the nurturing of the soul's relationships. In confronting real or imaginary threats to our existence or quality of life, discerning the difference requires a different orientation and view of how we fundamentally understand the world. Born into this world of generated existence, our character is tested repeatedly, and we experience the inevitability of suffering. The degree and term is largely determined by our own choice.

Our eternal nature remains carefully hidden behind a wall of our own fabrication, built upon a foundation of principles and values that reflect who and what we think we are. Yet, this is not what or who we are. If considered *desirable* and secondly *possible* for humanity to achieve a status worthy of mankind's place in the divine hierarchy, then it must involve inner contemplation, deep introspection, comprehension, and conscious self-awareness. Individuals and groups that are different than one's own need not represent an existential threat, but are in fact, necessary to promote a life in harmony by respect for others differences.

With the exception of a few, the vast majority of people remain rooted in the pathological character traits of the false-self. Largely unaware of tendencies suppressed by this personal Goliath—the principles of a quality of life worth living, of cooperation, collaboration, and genuine kindness and sincerity for others expressed in compassionate values worthy of our human species remain suppressed. Domination of one individual or group over another, clearly now recognized as undesirable, is abolished by radically altering the system that provides our physical, social and psychological needs. By reflecting values of cooperation and collaboration we sustain life-based principles worth living and avoid the narcissistic self-destruction that characterizes our preference for and reliance on the materialistic values of our modern age today. Too long now we have valued and sustained quantity over quality and emotional reaction to imaginary fear over conscious action towards a better life for all.

It is a high price we pay for ignoring this reality.

Until we recognize the monster in the mirror as ourselves, it remains elusive and undetected. Should we desire to confront and know our own suffering and misery, the creation by and of our own hands, it is found in the mirror of self-reflection. So, how do we create the impulse to know and face this? Does life continue to degrade to the point where we finally are compelled to seek the answers within us—a last ditch effort to save our own self?

Fundamental change about health-care will occur with a deeper understanding of ourselves and our true nature in relationship to each other. **This self-actualization comes from awareness, and only then will we actually care for and sustain one another, protecting ourselves against the *real* enemies of mankind—the old familiar two-headed Goliath-ego of ignorance and denial.** Understanding our position and role in the divine hierarchy—of a life of real meaning and purpose—begins with recognizing we are all souls that spring from the same universal source and share a common bond and ground in the sacred origin of life itself. This requires an understanding and knowledge that comes from *recognizing and remembering* who we are; our true heritage as the rightful heirs to the divine wisdom of our inheritance. Recognizing that we are ultimately responsible for our own destiny is difficult, and even more so harder to accept. Yet in time, all of this and more is revealed.

Short of a natural or man-made catastrophe, our current false-belief systems are likely to continue unless many, or at least a significant minority, evolve in this *self-awareness of the soul*. Our human tendencies derived from our social-political environment, exposed in the light of conscious-awareness, reveal the dark-side of the false-self ego. Embracing the evolution of individual consciousness, instead of suppressing it, means overcoming cultural socio-political factors by conscious and willful acts of intention by the individual. Changing first from within, then through active participation in newly developed behaviors, a new paradigm is created and manifested in our existence—a new world *deserving of a life worth living is re-born*. This is our birth-right.

Erich Fromm in 1973 summarizes this:

> *"None of these conditions are independent from each other. They are part of a system, and hence, reactive aggression can be reduced to a minimum only if the whole system as it has existed during the last six thousand years of history* <u>*can be replaced*</u>

> *by a fundamentally different one. If this occurs, the visions that were Utopian with the Buddha, the Prophets, Jesus, and the humanist Utopians of the Renaissance will be recognized as rational and realistic solutions serving the basic biological program of man: the preservation and growth of both the individual and the human species."*

Our social dilemma is a derivative of collective social passions rooted in character traits of the false-self ego and expressed in social values as *narcissism*. Emphasis on vices posing as virtues are triggered and influenced by manipulation of our deepest instinctual fears and desires. A clever age-old trick, this form of self-deception leaves us virtually powerless and vulnerable to falsely stimulated instinctual impulses. These are easily manipulated by the external authority-obeisance-submission model behind the illusion as *necessity*. Yet, to articulate and implement a new vision of human society based upon individual values and principles worthy of us remains undefined.

As the architects of the future, we either recognize as worthy a new life worth living in the 21st century based the values and principles of compassion and cooperation or continue the status quo of a malignant form of aggression characterizing the former. Mankind is in the act of re-creating itself, outside of itself. Careful consideration to the values and principles that reflect the best within us, will be of utmost importance.

We will remain indoctrinated by myths and superstitions if we do not follow the impulse for new dialogue about what we value as desirable for our future. Ideas and beliefs of our own creation underly the attitudes shaped by what we each value. If there is change to promote growth in our collective consciousness, it will begin with a reformed social character based on vastly different values and principles than that which persists under the current status quo.

Our victory over deeply rooted social-character passions of the false-self ego will ultimately be achieved in the unfolding and ascension of individual awareness: *the evolution of human consciousness of the soul's awareness of itself.*

Fromm:

"Human existence is characterized by the fundamental contradictions rooted in his physiological and psychical being: between his waning instincts and his growing self-awareness, a constant struggle to correct or compensate for the imbalance of separateness and powerlessness, of feeling "lost," and his desire to establish feeling home again in a world where he knows he doesn't belong."

This is the fundamental characteristic common to *all* people. However, it is satisfied *individually* in different ways, through affirming or destructive passions and emotions that we do *not* necessarily share in common with everyone; either love or hate, compassion or destruction, pride or humility, arrogance or humbleness, greed or charity, narcissism or altruism. We each express our actions and reactions differently in accordance to our particular level of awareness. The *key* to understanding this comes exclusively from neither the natural instinctive world nor the existential world of self-awareness.

In being devoted to a goal beyond his isolated ego, he ***transcends*** *himself and leaves the prison of absolute egocentricity.*

Mankind's destiny is largely achieved by our own hand. Efforts to establish new roots in the world provide a sense of belonging that is lost at physical birth and is experienced in growth. Aware of this separateness serves as motivation for the individual to create new ties to the world and to others through experiencing community and shared experiences. This frees us from the desperation of loneliness and powerlessness. The innate drive for fraternal community resolves mankind's dichotomous dilemma naturally. It restores his sense of unity, which is lost in self-awareness—the realization of being both in the seen and unseen worlds of the divine spirit.

The *identity* of the individual as one amongst many is crucial to our existence as a sovereign being. This identification with others as one's self is critical, as effectiveness in contributing to the well-being of the whole is measured by this.

This discourse of why suffering exists from a plague such as Lyme, though it is extremely critical of the medical community recognizes that Lyme is a consequence of an affliction of the human spirit. But as with all such diseases, plagues and maladies, the ultimate cure rests not only in our hands but in the minds that direct those hands. This is not to say that diseases are "all in your head" but that the cure exists when we have clear thinking about the cause, the source, of the actual problem. There is perhaps no quick or easy answer, or any answer at all, to whether this can or should be corrected. But, whether there is an answer or not is beside the point. It demands each one of us to at least consider this issue, and by recognition, acknowledgement, and acceptance, decide for ourselves whether to languish in "what is *not*" or exercise the power of our birthright to recognize what "*is*." Whether this happens or not is up to us.

The great enemy of humanity—the two-headed Goliath of our false-self ego—exists as a guide to the truth about our condition. Its two heads—ignorance and denial—serve the greater purpose of awareness and ascension as the counterpart necessary for motivation of will, the will to achieve a higher existence perfected by adversity. Simple recognition of this goes far towards the kind of unity that promotes liberation from suffering. But division also has its place. Without it, there would be no unity. When one learns this lesson, the two become one again, two parts of the whole. The coincidence of opposites that characterize the great paradox of our existence is also its resolution. A most difficult concept to grasp, the inevitable unity appears to our senses as a dichotomy in front of our face throughout our lives—an ever-tantalizing reality of the eternal present.

Meditation, Awareness and Transcendence

"I was ever frantically climbing ladders to pluck a ripe fig from some exotic overhanging garden of the past."
—Henry Miller

Miller's quote stuck home, reflecting upon the long period of recovery during treatment. With the gradual return of reason and rhyme came the ability to think sequentially and the will to live once again. But most importantly, a new direction and reverence for exercising this rejuvenated will in a *new life* emerged from the rear-view mirror. With the recent experience still predominant, the road ahead was largely a blank canvass waiting to be painted. Ever higher views of consciousness emerged as a result of this long ordeal. This arduous journey through the labyrinth of treatment to new life finally conceded to the long-forgotten feeling of feeling "normal" in one sense, but completely different in another. A new appreciation for even the most mundane features of everyday life dawned gradually. Emerging from this ordeal slowly yielded to a second coming—a resurrection of sorts. It was as if "raised from the dead" to a new life, as Lazarus did—a second birth in a very literal sense; born again.

The return to normal gave the past experience an eerie nightmare-like quality, a dreadful series of dream-sequences, a surreal journey akin to the return of Odysseus or Rip Van Winkle after a hundred-year snooze. But most of all, it is the story of Job. A new personality and identity began to emerge and flourish, one free of possessions of the body and soul. A sense of freedom previously unrealized brought with it a new appreciation for things unseen and emphasis on personal values unrealized.

As in the story of Job, faith was tested, and life restored. Prevailing on Social Security Disability Income was a real blessing, not just for me but for those who had cared for me during the ordeal, both as Caretakers and Benefactors, who no longer had to shoulder that burden. I had my life back, my family, and the means to sustain it again, and the sun rose each morning, and the coffee tasted good. A new appreciation for simple joys, mostly unrecognized before, took many forms, not the least of which being the great gift of meditation. Retained as a secret gift from the ordeal, this practice continued to give back much more than put in, ten-fold—even one hundred-fold.

Lessons from studies and research during the final years of treatment and recovery were in monastic self-reflection, intense retrospection and inner contemplation. *Meditation*, used as a way of coping with the Lyme debacle, assumed its place in daily life—a reward for the journey overcome, a secret gift for having survived the ordeal. Learning to accept with humility and dignity what is most difficult, the treatment and suffering endured was necessary for redemption of the spirit to begin anew.

At first with meditation came inner silence. While lying down on the back porch for hours, listening to the birds, the wind through the leaves, the frequent advance and retreat of the daily thunderstorm—hours would go by without moving, barely breathing, just barely alive, and yet, alive inside to the fullest. The sanctuary of the inner world brought relief in stillness. After long hours of involuntary practice, remaining a little longer each time, eventually *life itself* became a meditation. Slowly witnessing the gradual transition from a subjective to an objective view of existence, and then back again, a most peculiar and exaggerated feeling of separation of mind and body occurred in reverse, a distinct awareness of being two separate and interdependent entities joined again in union. This method of transcendence, a condition or state of being that comprised an entirely new perspective, took on a wholly different view from a new vantage point. That vantage point had shifted. A gradual process, overcoming the loss of former identity gave a new lease on life, one promising liberation from bondage. Our purpose in this world, liberation of the spirit is the highest goal; the achievement of mankind, humanities gift to itself. We begin as our own worst enemy. The enemy we seek to destroy is the monster within.

Armed with this new perspective, the inner mind, now as the vehicle for maneuvering this world in a new direction, was firmly in control. It is difficult to say whether this new perspective would have emerged if this shift in consciousness had not occurred. Because of the ordeal, this new world continues to come into fruition—an unfolding, a blossoming of Becoming revealed at a deeper level. It is a world where the old ways of everyday life no longer apply in the same way, now irrelevant, subject to a new set of laws, principles and values. Completely relevant for a new and better life, a new life worth living emerged.

A period of sheer astonishment began during this re-emergence into a new life. Around the time about two years without any medication (since 2012), there began a distinct feeling of ascension of the spirit, to heights unknown before nor ever dreamed of. Within the journey through the labyrinth of despair began an embryonic journey of a spiritual nature that transcends normal everyday life. Excelling again in study and research of science and spiritual topics, the South Berkshire Research Institute began in May of 2013, dedicated to solutions for a 21st century global society. While immersed in meditation study, reading countless books, and the monastic life of inner contemplation, interests in music returned and with it a recording studio. It seemed that life again was being restored ten-fold. Realization of this great gift, *meditation*, a precious and rare awareness, the seed of potentiality in *everyone* is eternally waiting to be recognized, acknowledged and accepted.

Miller continues:

> *To come into full recognition, "...one must act as if the past were dead and the future unrealizable. One must act as if the*

next step were the last, which it is. Each step forward is the last, and with it a world dies, one's self included."

This destiny with Lyme disease is characterized as one of symbolic *spiritual* death, resurrection and redemption. Lyme became retrospectively the lamp post that shed light on the true path home, the path to a new life worth living, not due to chance, but by divine guidance and the gift of grace. There are no coincidences in life. Each of us live according to the forces of our own destiny, in accordance with the immutable laws of nature. This eventually leads all back to the realm of the Divine whence we began. The balancing forces of karma at work in everyone's lives casts its blessing on all with its lessons providing guidance and correction. Gently or forcefully guiding the will, it is a kind of "moral compass" to guide our decisions and actions. At first, its small voice can be heard in our conscience, if we should but choose to listen to it.

This is the essence of what we call life.

By this pendulum of necessity we continue to rise and fall, to decline in disgrace and begin again in new faith. This faith is more than simply belief in things unseen. It is a faith born of *intuition*—of a direct experiential knowledge of what is. This process never fails to provide all that is required of us to understand the grace, the blessing of the great gifts of the Divine within. Remaining just out of sight until summoned, we come to recognize and finally accept these simple truths as gifts of grace. We are transformed and reborn in a true sense and suddenly realize we never actually left the Kingdom in the first place.

In the end, many of our false-self values and principles are illusions at best, and deliberate deception at worst. Yet there is a reason for this. The apparent disharmony that rules our world of generated existence is necesssary for good reason. But reason ultimately fails us in the great paradox, the contradictions and conundrums comprising our typical everyday world. Through the method of *transcendence* a path for reconciliation emerges in our life. The apparent disharmony that rules our world of generated existence is this way for a reason: necessity. Inflicting a burden nearly too great to bear, the path of redemption becomes clear. Yes, suffering need not be the only path to liberation of the spirit, but acceptance alone. Acts of compassion, charity and good will, the better way, are expressions of thanks and gratitude for the gift of grace by those who recognize, acknowledge and accept it. These many gifts and blessings are freely given, and it is our responsibility merely to recognize and accept them, but also express these values and principles by living them.

Reflected in the world through a life of love, mutual respect, tolerance, forbearance, honor, gratitude and compassion, we pay our debt of karma one way or the other. Knowing this living spirit is the key.

Carl Jung describes this experience of the 'living spirit' in "*Modern Man In Search of a Soul*":

> *"Such experiences reward the sufferer for the pains of the labyrinthine ways. From this point forward a light shines through his confusion; he can reconcile himself with the warfare within and so come to bridge the morbid split in his nature upon a higher level.... Who are forgiven their many sins? Those who have loved much. But as to those who love little, their few sins are held against them... The living spirit grows and even outgrows its earlier forms of expression; it freely chooses the men in whom it lives and who proclaims it. This living spirit is eternally renewed and pursues its goal in manifold and inconceivable ways through the history of mankind. Measured against it, the names and forms which men have given it mean little enough; they are only the changing leaves and blossoms on the stem of the eternal tree... Man is never helped in his suffering by what he thinks for himself, but only by revelations of a wisdom greater than his own. It is this which lifts him out of distress."*

This suggests that freedom from the human condition of suffering is accomplished by evolution of consciousness; the expansion and ascension of human conscious-awareness. The path to liberation of the spirit is singular-in-essence, but two-fold in nature: by atonement through suffering and acts of compassion and good will. This is the recognition, acknowledgement and acceptance of the great gift of what is.

EPILOGUE:

As the Silent Epidemic Continues

May your journey reflect the Divine within.

We see behind the mysterious debacle of Lyme disease exists a much larger issue. Anticipating this dialogue as extremely difficult and controversial is noted, as often the ultimate truth that liberates us is not what we anticipated or expected.

Nurturing well-being in both the body and soul guides our spirit to final liberation in union with the Divine. If we are to achieve and maintain a holistic view and balance of nature and spirit, acknowledgement and acceptance of the polarity and harmony of opposites is a necessary step forward. From whence it comes does not have to be proven to be acknowledged. The truth of its nature is revealed as self-evident.

Recognition is pervasive in both the material and spiritual spheres of existence. Not so much learned as re-called, re-collected or re-membered, silence and contemplation through meditation and inner reflection reveal the mysteries we know intuitively but have somehow lost in the noise and distractions of everyday life. Development of inherent skills of inner contemplation slowly yet steadily reveals this dual nature of our existence. Focusing at first on the small voice inside resumes a primordial ancient dialogue with the Master within, the mystic presence appearing as a teacher, guru, the Guardian Spirit that resides within each of us. Every person born of the flesh has this inner voice, supplied with all the necessary tools to activate and nurture it.

The material-dialectic during our current epoch characterizes the struggle within, between the false-self ego and the Guardian Spirit, as it has in all times. Passivity in action and decision incurs a determined fate that is not our own. *Intentional* action based upon the inner Guardian's voice *transcends* our knowledge of the external world and frees us from the chains of ignorance and superstition. Representing the inner Garden that we are responsible for cultivating to the degree possible, consciousness in this sense is the method by which the soul experiences the sensual world—a manifestation of the divine in nature. The physical body as the vehicle for the soul comprises the five physical senses which enable experience of the physical world through perception. To achieve liberation from the false-self ego, the spirit is set free by the soul back to the Divine from when it came—the spiritual realm. This is our primordial Home.

The path to well-being is worn by the footsteps of the wandering soul,
by ascension of consciousness, guided by intuition,
practiced in transcendence and achieved through awareness.

This can be done. It happened for me. And it can happen for all of us.

In conclusion, the ultimate answers we seek are not to be found "out there" as we have been led to believe; these are found *within*. While we continue futile attempts to escape the consequences of living in the world of generated existence through myth and superstition, faith picks up where and when belief in the utterly futile is finally abandoned by reason. Faith in something greater than ourselves and the world we are born into, perhaps incomprehensible to our common senses and unknowable to our intellect, is present nonetheless. With this kind of faith comes an understanding on a transcendental level; a knowledge born of intuition and matured by experience. Life is no longer perceived as an inevitable fate ruled by chance, coincidence and circumstance. As long as there are false beliefs to cling to by the egocentric man, the many false-messiahs, the Lyme-plagues and death itself will relentlessly point us in the right direction. Not up, not down, not east, west, north or south, not everywhere and anywhere, but *inward*. Despite efforts of science and technology, the solution and cure we seek in the external world that would save mankind from suffering reside within each one of us, and that spirit continues to repeat silently in a roar to those who can hear it:

"You can't fool Mother Nature."

By now you have grasped the gravity of the situation with regards to "the lie to big to admit." It can't continue indefinitely. But how many more will be sacrificed in the meantime? Awareness sometimes occurs stealthily and slowly, as does the disease when undetected. But, eventually it will manifest completely in a way that can no longer be ignored.

Lack of awareness and denial are still the biggest obstacles to preventing the spread, misdiagnosis and mistreatment of Lyme, and the cause of needless suffering to the afflicted, including the ones who must care for them. Don't wait. Be responsible to yourself and for the benefit of all who know you. Get tested with the guidance of a Lyme-literate doctor, and if necessary, get long-term antibiotic treatment. You owe it to not just yourself, but your loved ones.

APPENDIX

Additional Interviews of Stephen Amsden

EXCLUSIVE INTERVIEW with Stephen Amsden: Overcoming Lyme Disease

The Lymester

Published on YouTube

May 18, 2015

Question: Your full name please?

Stephen Edward Amsden.

Question: Where were you born and raised?

Born in Providence, Rhode Island 1959, and raised in southern central New Hampshire through 1977, then to college in Hartford, Connecticut.

Question: Do you have any children?

Yes, two daughters.

Question: When did you find out you had Lyme?

January 10th, 2009, approximately.

Question: Do you still have Lyme?

It's unknown. It's too early to tell. I have discontinued antibiotics after 44 months as of November of last year, so it's been three months. I'm still struggling. The primary symptoms that still seem to be prevalent are fatigue and widespread pain. The neurological and psychological issues seem to have vanished. They're gone. So, it's a little too early to tell. I've only stopped taking supplemental medication for the last three weeks, and it's my understanding there will be some time before I'll actually be free of the influence of those meds as well, so it's just too early to say. I don't know yet.

Question: How long have you had this infection?

Since nineteen seventy-four. I don't know if it was a tick bite, although it could have been. There was nothing like a rash or anything that precluded it. (Ed. note - in retrospect, this could have likely been Bartonella.) It was a series of tick bites later on in the 90s that probably reintroduced a new form of the infection, so there was that period in the 1990s. There were ample opportunities to be bitten by ticks, and the likelihood of transferring the illness during that time would be very high. Well, the tick bite or not I'm not sure, but the first incident in 1974 was upon returning from vacationing in Cape Cod, Massachusetts which our family did every summer.

Question: What was your reaction when you found out you had Lyme?

A tremendous sense of shock and of relief at the same time. Knowing what it was a great revelation, and at first gave me great hope thinking that, ah, we now know what it is, now I can do something about it. Until I learned what I was really in for.

Question: Did anybody know you had Lyme disease at that point, did you tell anyone else, or did anyone else know?

Well, when I found out, other than my immediate family and a few close friends, that's the only contact I had with society to begin with, so, oh I wasn't like I was shouting it from the rooftops. There were only a few people who were really involved in my life at that time.

Question: How did other people react when you told them?

Perhaps mostly disbelief. Because it's not a visible condition to most people. It's mostly a disease of the inside, it's not something that manifests physically or externally only in the most severe symptoms. So yeah, that's why. When it's hard to believe, right, there is a tendency for people to think that you're a hypochondriac and a malingerer. Inexplicable psychological behavior that's inexplainable. A lot of people will look at it that way.

Question: Did you know about Lyme, or try finding out about whether you had it?

Yes, I had been tested twice before, and had come back with negative results, knowing now looking back, of course those test results were highly unreliable and could even be completely in error. So, the third test proved positive.

Question: What kind of diagnosis or misdiagnosis did you get from different doctors?

Well, the first one was in 1974 upon returning from our vacation and Cape Cod, Massachusetts. While weeding in the garden, nice hot summer day in July, I stood up and saw an orb underneath the tree about the size of a beach ball. It had light, all the colors of the light of the of the rainbow, shimmering, undulating, changing, and it appeared to be the presence of some type of superior intelligence, perhaps an "angel," and it floated across the driveway up over the house. As I watched it go, I fell back into a grand mal seizure. From that I was diagnosed with epilepsy, first in 1974. That was the first misdiagnosis. It went on from there into my early adulthood coming through in terms of psychiatric manifestation. So early on, there were psychiatrists involved, but there were various other specialists who became involved, mostly from the psychiatric side. There was fatigue, then there was unexplained pain, this eventually brought on not only the misdiagnosis of depression and bipolar disorder, but rheumatoid arthritis, and then finally fibromyalgia, which is like a combination of all of the above. But then there are a number of neurological and psychological disorders anywhere from something like Tourette's syndrome to memory, cognition problems, ADHD was another one...

Question: Pretty much everything in the book!

Yeah, they ran out of things to diagnose me with and then ran out of medications to prescribe me, so they basically gave up. And it was at this point of having the borderline personality disorder and dementia, things were getting a lot worse. It was then that I was cornered for the third time to get the test. Having already been tested twice before with negative results, I fought my mother at 49 years old, saying emphatically, 'I don't have Lyme, I have fibromyalgia!' I was comfortable with that diagnosis and I didn't have the strength to battle her, so I acquiesced, got the third test, and it came back positive for "old" Lyme.

Question: What kind of symptoms did you normally experience while having Lyme?

In the beginning it was the neurological issues like petit mal seizures, where there would be this kind of jerking movement or "brain-zap" that would occur frequently to the point of every five seconds, and sometimes multiple times, but I was young then and still pretty strong and healthy otherwise, so I tolerated it well. One of the other things was sensitivity to light. I found it to be bright outdoor, and was constantly wearing sunglasses. Aside from the psychological and psychiatric type issues dealing with self-esteem and bipolar depression, besides those I could have easily been misdiagnosed with Multiple Sclerosis where the muscles in the back of my legs were not working right, they were convulsing, sending convulsions or seizures to my head.

The other symptoms circulate around widespread pain, mostly joint pain in my arms, hands, wrists, fingers, knuckles; a profound fatigue, just a weakness where it made it difficult to get out of bed. Couldn't do anything. And a type of dementia where the faculties that we normally consider make us human, like will, reason, the emotions, those are gone, they're not there anymore. You start to question whether you are really even human anymore. So, there could have been a number of other misdiagnoses. I could have had Parkinson's due to the tremors that I was having, I was misdiagnosed ADHD, unable to focus, to concentrate, couldn't read anymore, so the psychiatric issues, the widespread pain, the fatigue, and a crippling anxiety, a fight or flight syndrome that was overpowering, and the feeling of being slowly suffocated, like I was drowning, couldn't get enough air. Those four things - the psychiatric issues, widespread pain, debilitating anxiety, and chronic fatigue - those are the four pillars for most of the manifestations of Lyme.

Question: So, you were having issues physically and mentally at this point?

Yeah, it pretty much involved everything at that point, and there could be multiple symptoms ranging from one side to the other depending on which day. There was no rhyme nor reason to it, there was no pattern, there was nothing that I could associate with what was going on that would cause this kind of thing. it seemed to be totally random.

Question: You must have been feeling desperate at this point.

You reach a point of desperation and then you go beyond that.

Question: What was actually the hardest part of dealing with this?

The hardest part is being cut off from humanity, being in a state of solitary confinement, and this feeling that you just don't belong, you do not belong, period. That's the hardest. Depersonalization, the loss of identity, who you are. It's like being trapped inside a dirty terrarium that you can't get out of, and you're watching life go on outside of it, and you're stuck on the inside, alienated. But it is the dementia part of it that is definitely the worst - the worst.

Question: Very interesting how Lyme can affect people in so many different ways, some people have mainly physical symptoms and with other people psychological. What would you say is necessary to treat and cure the disease, such as when it comes to not being covered by health insurance, one has to pay for all or most of it, and most doctors won't touch a Lyme patient. How were you able to handle that, how were you able to find help, where did you go to?

To combat late-stage, disseminated 'old' Lyme it's usually necessary for a long-term protocol of powerful antibiotics. This has been demonstrated over time again and again with the majority of patients as the best choice for combating the disease, and has demonstrated being effective in terms of improving overall the Lyme patients capabilities and their ability to enjoy life, the quality of life. So, you have to find a Lyme-literate doctor (LLMD) who is capable and willing to administer long-term antibiotic protocols, not just for a period of days or weeks, but months, and possibly years for the advanced cases. So, finding a Lyme-literate doctor is number one, but finding one who is essentially going to see you through to the finish line, that's essential.

Question: This runs counter to the prevailing attitude that if you've been treated for 30 days, you're done, you're cured, you don't need anything else. I mean, it's a doctor, so you kind of feel like your supposed to listen to them, they're supposed to know more than you, right?

Yes, but this is often not the case. Your average family physician is often less informed than the patient they are treating. Notice I say treating, not healing. And, the length of time it takes for recovery can easily lead one to believe that the protocol is not working, and this is the counter-intuitive part of treatment, that typically you would think that with a long-term antibiotic protocol that you would start to feel better. But it's not the case. In actuality, you feel much worse due to the die-off of the bacteria leaving behind toxins which cause inflammation throughout the body, so it's a fairly miserable process of recovery. And it is likely that the number one reason that people relapse is that their doctors do not prescribe a long enough course of antibiotics to make it to the finish line. But on the other hand, often the patient is unable to endure the side effects of recovery they are so severe. There's a lot going against someone who has it. So, there are two things going against you even if you know that you have the disease:

1) Finding a Lyme-literate doctor who is experienced and knowledgeable, and will keep you on a protocol it long enough to get you well again;

2) You are a patient who is resilient and persistent, consistent and unfaltering in your application of that antibiotic protocol. Yes, it is ultimately your responsibility for becoming well. All a good LLMD can do is give you the tools and means to get there; the rest is up to you.

Question: It's rather similar in some ways to cancer.

There are some people who have Lyme who would gladly trade it for almost any other type of cancer. As a matter of fact, there was one Lyme patient who was excited at the knowledge that she had cancer, because she thought that finally she was going to get the protocol that would get rid of the Lyme. That's how desperate some Lyme victims are.

Question: What do you feel is the best way to optimize one's chances of triumphing over this disease?

To optimize your chances of survival, it could be necessary that you have a caretaker, an advocate as well as your Lyme-literate doctor. The caretaker being that if you are in a situation where the symptoms are so severe that you are unable to work, and in my case, I was unable to do anything, a kind of paralysis, then the caretaker role may have to be taken up by someone else. If you cannot care for yourself during that time, yes, it's going to increase your chances or your probability success if you have a caretaker. And now if you have an advocate, that's someone who will look after your affairs, make sure that you get to the doctor bills paid on time, that you're going to be able to afford to maintain, to perhaps live with while not working. You have bills to pay, there are a lot of expenses involved, so how does one afford the treatment when you are unable to work? Well, that's the advocacy part. An advocate is someone who is going to basically provide financial assistance and otherwise other physical means of getting you through this time, be it the weeks, months or years that it might take. This could be a family member, friend, or even a support group. There's only going to be a small percentage of people who have the good fortune to be in that situation where they have a caretaker and an advocate. It may be necessary in order to beat the disease, and if you don't have that, well that certainly decreases your probability of getting to the finish line. Unfortunately, most won't.

Question: Why do you think it is so hard to prevail over Lyme?

Probably because it goes undetected for so long. It often starts off with very mild symptoms early on that can persist for years before getting worse, or you may be administered other medications that suppress the symptoms and allow it to continue to fester and to permeate your body. And a lot of your own defense mechanisms, just as a human being will help compensate for detriment from either the physical or psychological effects, you may find ways of dealing with it. And, the psychiatric medication certainly suppresses the symptoms, meanwhile, as these symptoms are being suppressed, the source of the disease is flourishing until you're at a point where you're in a crisis situation and everything you've done before doesn't work anymore. You suddenly find yourself where you're unable to cope with your existing situation. What I've noticed the most in coming out of this debacle is in looking around and the awareness of how widespread this disease is, and to what extent.

There is a whole generation of children being born with the disease to mothers who unknowingly carry the infection. Now, how many generations will it be if this goes undetected before we as a species will be unable to produce viable offspring? That alone is essential that we come up with some answers, and quickly. Now, that's one of the more disturbing realizations coming out of this, how widespread it is, and these young mothers who are unknowingly passing the disease to their unborn child. So, let's just say, for instance, for the sake of this example that one out of ten people end up having the disease. Of those one out of ten, you put all those people in that group, and one out of ten of that group will actually find a LLMD who can deal with their situation. So you take the one out of ten from that group, and you have a new group. Now this group, one out of ten of those will actually stay with a protocol long enough to make a meaningful difference in their lives, and out of those people, one out of ten of them will actually make it to the finish line due to their own resilience and perseverance. So, the chances of recovering or the probability of recovering are very small. The one out of ten out of ten out of ten... I mean, it just gets to a smaller and smaller group of people who actually have a chance of making it, and this is what I would call the 'chosen ones'.

The chosen ones for whatever reason, be at their own genetic disposition, by absolute just plain dumb luck of finding out that you've got it and not something else, finding a doctor who can treat it, and will treat you long enough, and if they're willing to treat you long enough, can you stand the severity of the symptoms of treatment long enough. So, it's up to the doctor, but it's ultimately up to you as the patient whether you have the resilience to get far enough. It's kind of like being stuck in a swamp. If you do nothing, you go no further, and you sink. Once you start through that swamp, don't stop. You're taking an antibiotic protocol that is propelling you through the swamp; you keep going, no matter how long it takes. It's different for everybody, it could be weeks for some, months for another, years for some others, it depends on how long you've had it, what number of co-infections you may have had with it, but you do not stop. Once you make that journey, until you get to the other side. It is very Darwinian. There's only going to be a few who are going to survive. A lot of variables.

Question: Also, your advocate and caretakers are somebody that to keep you on that path, right, when you're in that type of a situation you can't do it on your own. It's kind of its like expecting a drug addict to get off the drug by himself.

That's right, it's where it was an intervention. I was 49 years old and my mother had to intervene on my behalf, because I was unable to. Who else was going to? There was nobody else. Are there any other people that you know that had Lyme they're closed to you?

Yes, my youngest daughter Leah, my youngest brother Randall. My father had babesia last summer, has been bitten numerous times, as a land surveyor has been for 50 years, how can he not have it? It's almost impossible not to get it in our situation. Some of the myths about it being 'hard to catch' and 'easy to cure' is utter nonsense. It's been proved over and over - there is so much anecdotal evidence to the contrary, it's easy to get and it's hard to get rid of. These are two of the myths that have been propagated for years, and why they still have any credibility, or do they? It's unbelievable.

Leah has made it across the finish line and is in the "wait-and-see" period where you see if there is going to be any relapse, or time will tell. there's only so much you can do now but wait and see. And my youngest brother Randall, he has prevailed on Social Security disability. He is completely disabled. He's been on and off protocols now for several years, and could still be very much afflicted and very much struggling with the disease.

Question: Why do you think it has been so difficult for him to overcome it?

The same reason of it taking so long to be diagnosed. He's probably had it for 20 years or more, and of course we're led to believe it was because of this or that or anything except what it was, so by the times you're completely disabled, it becomes almost impossible to get rid of it. Although most everybody shows remarkable improvement, there's still only a few who are actually going to make it through across the finish line, so…

Question: If I think I might have Lyme, even though I don't know how it might have been possible, what would be your best advice?

Find out whether you have it or not. If everybody made that choice, everybody would find out whether they're a carrier. If there's something you can do about it now before it becomes a crippling affliction, then there may be a chance of avoiding the labyrinth that the rest of us have fallen into and find it so hard to get out of. So, certainly find out now before the symptoms become so prevalent that you're looking for any answer. And when you're driven by desperation, you're more apt to accept the wrong conclusion, the wrong diagnosis, so calmly going about finding out for sure whether those pains in your muscles and joints, is it just "getting older" as I was told for years, or is there actually something there? Well, it may be so mild that it's not preventing you from going to work, from thinking, or doing or whatever it is, but certainly finding out to be sure now before it gets you later when it's too late, that's probably the best thing we can do as a species in a society where we impact each other. So, awareness and then the desire to find out for sure whether you are a carrier, that's probably the best thing that you can do for yourself, for your loved ones, and for society in general.

The difficulty with the testing, to nail down whether for sure it's the case with you or not, that is the big issue. The current standards for testing in your common labs has a dreadful failure rate of false negatives, where you could be tested for it and it comes back negative, and yet you find out down the road that, oh no, you have full-blown Lyme for the last three years. Well, why didn't they catch it, you know, three years ago when you first got tested? Well, the tests are notably erroneous, and aside from one lab in Palo Alto, California called IGeneX (they use a combination of tests that claim to have a ninety-five percent accuracy rate). It was not until I got tested through IGeneX; it was then that I learned that in fact I did have the Lyme.

I had tested twice for before, and had come back negative, so those negative test results propelled me for another seven or eight years of further becoming infected. And thinking that all the while that 'well it can't be Lyme, I've been tested twice - it was negative both times,' it just was not the case. If you test negative it does not mean you do not have Lyme. So, when you decide to find out, use IGeneX. If you're going to find out for sure, you do not want to use these labs which two out of three are coming back with the wrong results. It's not that it won't help you, it's even worse than that - it's just going to make things so much worse. So, that's the thing about the test. IGeneX. There are tests that are coming out now that are supposedly more accurate. It will come, but don't wait until then. The time to find out is now."

***

EXCLUSIVE INTERVIEW with Stephen Amsden: Chronic Lyme Disease, A Global Threat

The Lymester/Shift Happens Project

The Lymester

Published on Nov 20, 2015

Advanced late stage chronic Lyme Disease as a global threat is discussed in detail in this riveting dialogue between Sparke Carrier (Shift-Happens Radio) and Stephen Amsden (The Lymester).

Question: So, let's get back to business here now. We're going to talk about Lyme disease today. Now when I met Stephen a couple years ago, I was aware at the time that he had Lyme disease or had experienced it. And I don't want to say 'survivor' because I don't like that terminology, you are a creator and an informer, so I just would like to first off welcome Stephen Amsden. Stephen, welcome to the show here.

Thank you, it's good to be here.

Question: I'm so glad you're here, because you've got lots of information that you can share with people. The best thing that we could do to start out is I have some questions: When did you actually get Lyme disease, do you know?

When I was 15 years old, this is in 1974, our family usually each year during the summer went to Cape Cod for a week or two for vacation, and we had just returned from our regular vacation on the Cape. It was probably about the end of June beginning of July, was hot and I was working in the garden with my parents and my brothers. We were all out there weeding the garden, it was hot, and I stood up and everything turned silvery. I was not right in the head and at first I thought well, it's just the heat, but I decided I would sit down and get a drink of water and my parents agreed. They said go ahead, and I walked down the path of the garden, and everything was turning silver, just this surreal kind of background, and underneath the maple tree at the east of the garden I saw a glowing ball of light that was about the size of a beach ball, perhaps a little larger, maybe three feet in diameter, and all of the colors of the rainbow were shimmering and shining, changing and undulating in it. And I pointed it out and exclaimed "Look, look!" It was like being in the presence of some type of superior intelligence, it was 'otherworldly' and at first because of my background I thought this is God, you know, this is God, and then it occurred to me after a few seconds of observing this seemingly intelligent sentient being that well, perhaps it was a messenger from God, it was an angel, and at that time it started floating across the driveway and up over the roof of the house. And as my eyes followed it, it was so overwhelming, I fell back into a grand mal seizure. I was so overwhelmed by the sensation of encountering this phenomenon that I woke up on the ground, and the dog was looking right in my face.

So now, upon that happening, of course, the day after I ended up going to the hospital for some routine tests. They tested me and came up with a diagnosis of "epilepsy," so I had these kind of slight trigger events in my mind, just like a camera shutter going off periodically and randomly, like these little brain zaps, little jolts, and so is their diagnosis, and they put me on a huge bottle of pills that look like the Tower of Babel sitting in the middle of the kitchen table. Three times per day of Dilantin (an anti-convulsant). Well, that was the beginning of my journey, and I could easily wrap it up and say, well, you know, just refer to the story of Job and there you'd have it, but I will for the sake of brevity go over the history of this, because I think being misdiagnosed so many times over the years are a telltale sign of Lyme, and what many people go through when it's undetected.

So, it started off I was just teenager at 15 years old. I had to postpone getting my license at 16 years old for another year and had to go two years without having another seizure on the Dilantin. And the doctors were, 'well, it could be that it will resolve on its own and it'll never happen again' and it never did. However, I went out on through my later teenage years, went to college, early adult life, got married, got a job, had children and at about 28 years old, I was having some difficulty with depression, and yes, this was my second misdiagnosis. Now it had been let's see about 12-13 years that I basically just lived with the little trigger events going on in the mind, but also now having issues with depression which wasn't uncommon. I was under a lot of pressure; did not seem excessively abnormal under the circumstances, so I did take some medication, Librax, an anti-anxiety med, but I discontinued that after a couple of years. We moved to New Hampshire and at that time I was also under a lot of pressure due to the move, so this is several years later again coming back on the depression medication.

Now I was able to basically overcome that for another six or seven years until it returned again in the 1990s. This time we were in the middle of another move, and there was a lot of pressure, and again the this time it was diagnosed as *manic depression.* I took Serzone (the SSRI Nefazodone) for seven years very successfully. It did a great job suppressing the symptoms, and I had probably the most productive years of my life in terms of career advancement, being a father, playing in a band, I was very involved and effective. So, we're coming up now on the late 1990s and as I became more successful, there was also more pressure and the demands of the medication to suppress the depression were increased repeatedly, so I was prescribed additional medication. And this continued to suppress the symptoms but in reality permitting the actual cause to flourish, until in the early 2000s I was succumbing to this chronic anxiety that was just overpowering. I'd have these panic attacks that I could not suppress with the anti-depressants, and the effort to suppress this was not working anymore. I went back. I was diagnosed this time with *chronic anxiety disorder.*

A lot of that was psychiatric in the beginning, epilepsy being a kind of a neuro-degenerative thing way back was an indicator. Right now, with the chronic anxiety I was taking Lorazepam and this did wonders for that, again suppressing the symptoms, and I'll say now that no one along this journey as far as any of the doctors ever tried to really find out what was wrong with me. I came back to them with the symptoms again and again, they just gave me the medication, bat it back down, and that was it. That was the game we were in now. Anxiety was being controlled, but it was getting worse, requiring greater doses in higher doses of Clonazepam and increasing the dosages and number of other anti-depressants. I started developing a condition of ADD or ADHD, kind of like an adult version. Well, I had the anxiety disorder, but the inability to focus and concentrate was becoming an issue, so I was prescribed Adderall, an amphetamine. They did their best with marvelous substances to suppress the symptoms, but it came to a point where I was on like seven or eight different meds, a cocktail of pharmaceuticals that were no longer working. Well, they couldn't come up with enough to keep me going anymore at that point, and I was failing in my career, my job, everything was suffering from it. I was forced to resign in 2006 after a 25-year career in high-tech, as I could no longer do the job, and I was in trouble. I had rental properties and a lot of responsibilities, my home, my children, and I was trying desperately to recreate myself. I moved to Florida, changed my job. I worked on a bamboo farm, a complete turnaround, complete contrast to my previous life, but it was a little late. It was an attempt to recreate myself because I was having terrible identity issues. My identity was gone. I was no longer the person that I used to be, and I'm sure there were parts that were missing that were part of my personality, that I was no longer the same person.

Question: So, when you lost all of that, would you say that was more because of the drugs, or was it about the disease itself?

It was the underlying disease itself. The reason I went as long as I did was because of what the pharmaceuticals that they were supplying me with. So, they did their best to keep me going under terrible circumstances. I did about seven or eight months on the bamboo farm where I did have this great kind of a rebirth, but it was over very quickly. With all the pharmaceutical still in place after seven or eight months, I ended up going to a doctor with severe physical pain in the joints - my arms, wrists, all over really, my whole body, but mostly in my arms. My arms felt like they were being electrocuted. I felt like I had my fingers stuck in an electrical outlet. It was really torturous, 24/7. The pain never went away, and for the first time, this general practitioner actually tried to find out what was wrong with me and ran probably 30-40 tests on all he could think of. I did demand a Lyme test at this point as part of the testing that he did, and he wanted that, but all he came up with was a slight indicator that I might have some type of rheumatoid arthritis. Then he recommended me to a Rheumatologist. He ruled out the rheumatoid arthritis, and he diagnosed me with *fibromyalgia*. This is the garbage bucket for people like myself who don't fall into one of these other neat little categories or diagnoses, and I also demanded a second Lyme test, which of course came back negative. Okay, this is one of the issues with testing. The false negatives that come back from your common labs like Labcorp, these are just notoriously inaccurate. So, they missed it twice with a bad test. Instead, they came up fibromyalgia, my final misdiagnosis.

Now on my way to disability, I got a lawyer, lost all my properties, got foreclosed, declared bankruptcy, got divorced - basically I lost everything. And this is the story of Job. This is where I basically lost everything including my health, identity... I went to my lawyer and I said 'look, I'm either headed for prison, the nursing home, or at the end of the road' and he did help me. It took two years to become officially disabled. I did prevail on that in the end, but I was in no better shape. I was worse.

I was getting worse, and this is where I remember talking to my parents - I was still living in Florida at the time. I mentioned to them that I didn't know how much longer I could continue to take care of myself, and my mother insisted that I come up to New Hampshire to get re-tested for Lyme. I argued with her, I was like 'mom, I don't have Lyme, I've already been tested twice. I don't have it, I have fibromyalgia, leave me alone!' I just didn't have the strength to battle her over it, and I reluctantly agreed, went up and got tested. And I remember telling this doctor, a Lyme-literate doctor, "You know, if my mother is right, I'm going to build a shrine to her!" And after explaining my long-term symptoms, the doctor said, 'well you better start saving your money for that shrine because I'm ninety-five percent certain that you have late-stage advanced Lyme disease.'

When I got the tests back, that's exactly what it was - she says 'You have 'old' Lyme. It's advanced. You've had it for years and years, and I thought at the time it was quite a revelation. I'll never forget that moment when I found out. It's one of those ah-ha moments in life where I thought, well, maybe this is good. I don't have fibromyalgia. I don't have this long torturous kind of near death sentence that's just going to linger, until I found out later about the reality of Lyme. And then it's a toss-up! Which would be worse, I don't know, but at least with Lyme I figured, okay, there's at least a chance I can be cured. Well, how little of a chance that was going to be was not known at the time, and how I might have got it at Cape Cod being bitten by a tick. We were out in the tall grass playing around, me and my brothers, and it's very likely I picked up a deer tick. It may have been a co-infection like babesia or bartonella, or ehrlichia, those are related co-infections that often come with Lyme, and that perhaps in my later years I may have picked it up again. I don't know on that, it's impossible to say, all I know is that the symptoms that I had back when I was 15, I don't have anymore as a result of the treatment.

So, when I look at exactly what it did it take to call myself *cured*, as of now I've been completely antibiotic free for almost two years, and medication and pharmaceutical free completely for two years. So, for the first time in my adult life, I never knew that it was possible to feel this good. In other words my whole life I was suffering with whatever it was, to me that was normal. I mean, I never knew anything different, So, the past two years have been what most people would refer to as "normal." There is such a thing as normal, and for Lymers it's called the "promised land," and that's where I've been for the past two years.

Question: Okay, that's excellent. Two years is a long time. Can you give us some of the common myths now, we know that they you were misdiagnosed with fibromyalgia and previously with depression, etc. but were there other possibilities that they were looking into when they were diagnosing you, when they were testing you, that they were naming as possibilities?

Well yes, in a way, the rheumatoid arthritis misdiagnosis kind of led to the fibromyalgia misdiagnosis. But in looking back, I could have easily have been misdiagnosed with multiple sclerosis, Parkinson's, ALS, Alzheimer's, lupus, the whole host of neuro-degenerative diseases, any of these by just going to the "right" specialist. They call Lyme the 'great imitator' because it has over 300 symptoms that can be associated with these other diseases. These other chronic illnesses, however, I think this is one of the myths about Lyme, that it is not an 'imitator,' it is the 'Originator,' that these chronic illnesses are manifestations of Lyme disease. This is what's the tragedy of what's happening; people are frequently being misdiagnosed with these chronic illnesses and they never actually find out the source of it. They treat the symptoms, and the person just degenerates into a living hell, and that's exactly what happens.

There is a much larger picture involved with the medical community in general that ignores this problem, and there are many reasons for this, but none of them are good, so yeah, there are so many misdiagnoses that can happen you'll never actually get to the source itself. Which, in my experience, and what I see is so widespread is that people just are not aware of this yet, and I say yet. When they do find out what's going on, we will find out so many people will have suffered and died unnecessarily. It's just it's an enormous tragedy, the cost, incalculable.

Question: What did it actually take for you to become cured?

The first thing to getting cured is that you have to be tested successfully, and there is one lab out in California called IGeneX. Now IGeneX has a a double test that has a ninety-five percent accuracy rate, and this is far above your common labs which have a notoriously poor track record in terms of accuracy. Your typical labs will maybe four out of ten tests will show false negative results, so the main thing is to get tested at IGeneX. When I got that test, this is the third test, I had what showed as positive.

Now when you have a positive diagnosis, you need to find a Lyme-literate doctor (LLMD) and this will be an infectious disease specialist who is knowledgeable about Lyme and has treated people successfully. They are a rare breed; you're not going to find easily a Lyme doctor, they do not have neon signs over their offices saying "We do Lyme!" No, they pretty much have to keep hidden and stay under the radar. It's more like trying to get an abortion in a back alley in the 1950s, so it's hard to find them. They do exist, though, through advocacy groups like Lymedisease.org, where you can find one of these doctors. Now a good Lyme literate doctor is going to look at the long-term symptoms based upon your current information. If this doctor says 'oh, you can be easily cured in 30 days,' this is probably just not true, especially for a late stage advanced Lymer. I remember my doctor leveling with me right off saying 'you know, it's going to take many, many months of treatment to bring you back, perhaps years,' and this is how long it did take.

Once an antibiotic protocol was prescribed, clarithromycin, doxycycline, and plaquenil, these are three very powerful drugs. One is an anti-parasite, the other two go after the bacteria, and it took almost four years – 44 months. During that time, the treatment is absolutely miserable, and this is counterintuitive. This is why so many people who start, even if they have the test results, they have the right doctor, they have the right protocol, the fourth obstacle is the *duration of treatment.* Most people can't handle the symptoms of treatment. Typically, we think when we take antibiotics, well, we start feeling better, it's such a relief. Not so with Lyme. With Lyme, you actually feel much, much *worse,* and you're already pretty bad off to begin with. It's actually the die-off of the bacteria releases toxins, which causes inflammation in the body's tissues. It is called a "Herx reaction," which can come and go with some people, but for me it was like a three year ordeal on the couch, paralyzed, unable to move, unable to think, just this dreadful kind of not even what I would call actually *living,* it was just *existing.* You don't have your human faculties. I remember screaming at my doctor "Am I even human anymore?" I had no reason, no empathy, no will, no determination anymore, anything. Your gone.

So, you're in this chronic anxiety, chronic fatigue state, crippled and just in this terrible place where I needed a caretaker. I depended upon my parents at 45 years old. Back to depending on my parents: it's all very humiliating, but in looking back, I mean, that's all nonsense. You have to do what you have to do. *You can't let money get in the way.* None of your insurance is likely to pay for it, as **the medical community does not recognize chronic Lyme disease as a true illness**. But you cannot let money get in the way. For someone to say 'Well, I can't afford to get treated for Lyme,' well, you can't afford *not* to, because it's so debilitating that I spent months just wondering why am I even trying, you know, I might as well just get it over with. And suicide is a very prevalent problem with advanced late stage Lymers who are in treatment, or not in treatment. So, I had to deal with that, and thank goodness I had a supportive family and friends and people who cared enough so that if I weren't around, they'd be miserable. That kept me going. It was like, okay I'm not going to do it for me, but I'll do it for them, and thank goodness I did, you know, because when you finally come out of it on the other end, oh, life is better than you ever could have imagined. So yeah, 44 months for me before I started feeling better, and it still takes a while after that. My doctor was upfront with me and told me, "well, your neuro symptoms could last for up to a year after you're cured," and that's exactly what happened.

Question: What were some of the obstacles that you actually experienced?

The biggest obstacle is *awareness*. And we talked a little, but about that with the insurance companies not wanting to pay for this long-term treatment, so there's a concerted effort to suppress information about Lyme. And that's why we don't know much about it still, even though it's been around for 40+ years and is claiming more and more victims every year, in terms of hundreds of thousands, so that's one of the obstacles. The other is the scarcity of Lyme-literate doctors (LLMDs), and there's your concerted effort to prevent people from taking long-term antibiotics. You'll hear this in the press, they'll say, 'oh, we are overusing antibiotics and is creating these superbugs that are resistant.' Well, that may be true, but that's more propaganda to squash the knowledge about Lyme and what it takes to recover from it. Those are some of the main obstacles, but there are many others also.

If you have symptoms that are anything from sleep deprivation to aches and pains, they could seem relatively minor, but you're being brushed off by your general practitioner, or you're being given medication just to suppress the symptoms, trust your instincts, trust your body and what your body is telling you and pursue it. If I had found out so much earlier on, my life would have been so much different, perhaps much better, so I have a hard and fast law that I propose to people, and that is:

"Don't rule out Lyme until Lyme has been ruled out."

That's the law that I would lay out before people if I could. And they're is a close corollary, and that is to that is *do it first*. It's one thing to want to be tested, but you don't want to wait until you've been tested for everything else, because they'll misdiagnose you into things that will keep you going for 20 or 30 years before you find out. This is one of my big mistakes. Now, I did try to find out early on, I did get the test, but I got it at the wrong place.

Question: We have a health care system that, let's face it, first of all, the doctors, I mean, there's just so much pressure to get people in and out, and it's about getting pushed by pharmaceutical companies as well. And here, you can take these, and you can pass those out, and we'll pay you this much money if you can turn around and start incorporating this or that. And it's not just in the doctor offices, it's in the school system, it's the same thing, so of course they would rather see a sick society than a well society.

Right. Yes, that's right, this is endemic of the larger picture, this is the larger issue. It's not just Lyme, it's cancer, it's all of the diseases. They're all making money from it and certainly seeing someone cured, well, our whole system is not geared to that, so there are many to accept the blame. The blame can be shared by amongst many, that's part of the problem.

Question: And again the fact that ignorance on the part of the medical industry when it comes to the disease itself, not knowing. Or worse, ignoring the evidence while at the same time denying its existence and that information about the symptoms, doctors in general are not educated well enough.

That's exactly right, yes, they are not told about it. They might receive a 15-minute briefing in a medical journal about Lyme, but even infectious disease specialists typically are woefully ignorant of Lyme and its many, many manifestations, and how to treat it. This is where your Lyme-literate doctor is essential to making it to the finish line. If you go to an infectious disease specialist who does not know about Lyme, they may give you one month of antibiotics and forever after consider you cured, no matter what your symptoms are after that. And this is what they've been told, is what they've been taught, and where that's coming from, well, that's probably another conversation for another night, for sure.

Lyme can be transferred via other avenues than the tick. This typically is the one method people are aware of, which is one of the lingering myths that you can only get Lyme from a tick. While this is true that the tick probably remains the primary means of transmission into the human body, however, we know now there are a total of four known ways, the tick bite being the most well-known. But less well known is that the public blood supply can become infected unknowingly when someone gives blood, you could go in to get surgery in a hospital anywhere in the United States, or in the world for that matter, and become infected through transfusions. The third way we know about, and this is the biggest tragedy of all, I think, and that is young mothers who are unknowingly infected who are unknowingly giving or passing the disease to the fetus during pregnancy. So, we have a whole generation of children who are being born with the disease, and this could manifest as autism, your ADHD or a ADD diagnosis in children, obsessive-compulsive disorder, juvenile arthritis, which my youngest daughter was misdiagnosed with when she was five. So, this is a huge tragedy.

There are all of these young mothers who are just not aware that they have it, that they've passed it to their children, so this is the third way we know of. And now the kicker, here is the clincher. The fourth way is that it can be transmitted sexually. It is actually a spirochete very similar to syphilis, and in fact, you could almost consider the Borrelia spirochete possibly as a genetically modified organism based upon syphilis, perhaps a distant "cousin." Now, I don't know that for certain, but this is all good material for perhaps another conversation about it. That's another whole area about whether borrelia was weaponized back in the 50s and 60s, and I often wonder if I was part of some kind of bio weapon warfare experiment way back there in the seventies. So yeah, one thing about getting it by sexual transmission, and if that's the case, then we can expect probably a majority of the population to have it if they don't already. So, that's the reality of it, but you won't hear about this through the mainstream media.

Question: Of course not.

Right. You're only are going to find this by doing your own research, and I encourage anyone who's concerned about this, and everybody should be, so do your research, get on Google, get on YouTube, start looking under those stones and turning over those stumps and digging out that information, because you're not going to get it from your doctor. You're not going to get it from the medical community. So, here we are.

Question: Wow. That's amazing. I thought there was only one way to get it, being bitten by a tick.

That's still one of the several big myths about Lyme. They say, 'oh, it's hard to get and easy to cure,' well no, it's not. That's a misleading statement. It's *easy* to get, and it can be *difficult* to cure. If you catch it early, yes, you can cure it easily. Right. But, it's so easy to miss and be misdiagnosed that you go beyond that 30 days and you're in a heap of trouble. So, that's one of the big myths. Probably the biggest one.

We have talked about awareness. It is slowly becoming more available to people. The information. I would recommend that anyone who thinks that they themselves or a family member or a friend or someone they know, if they think they might have the symptoms that indicate Lyme, I would recommend seeing the video *"Under Our Skin."* It's a little dated now, it's what, seven or eight years old, but it's still a very viable documentary. It is very eye-opening, and they just came out with a sequel to it called "*Emergence*" intended as a follow-up. Those two videos are extremely important for anyone who is interested in learning more, or like I said, that may exhibit some of these symptoms, or they see it in their children. I would start there, you will be astounded at what you'll learn just from those two. Those are like the gold standard for documentaries on Lyme. When you come to understand the full extent and how far it's come, it is astounding what we still don't know about it. But like I said, it is starting to get out there, and it's through programs like this and people talking about it that we're going to get the word out.

Question: You've shared an absolutely incredible message tonight, something that is well worth everyone taking the time to listen to, so I'm going to make a point that we share this video as much as possible, because this information is important for everyone to hear and know. So, I thank you again, Stephen, you just absolutely rock this planet. I thank you so much for taking the time and, also I know you've done the research. You've not only experienced it, you've gone beyond and found the cure for yourself, and in doing that, what you're doing is opening the doors for other people to go and be cured themselves as well. Thank you for joining the Shift-Happens Radio Show Stephen.

I'm pleased to do it. Thank you, thank you so much.

***

MEET THE AUTHOR

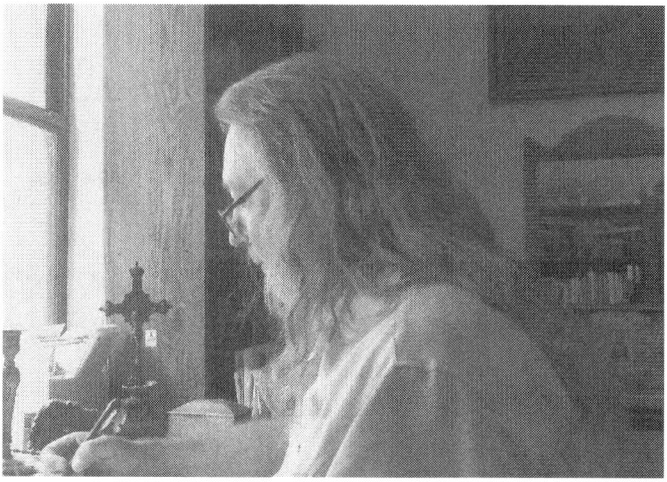

Stephen Edward Amsden, Rosicrucian, Martinist, Theosophist, is founder of the South Berkshire Research Institute of Spiritual Science and the Lymester Advocacy Group. Stephen majored in Philosophy at the University of Hartford, receiving a Bachelor of Science in Computer Science from Franklin Pierce College after employment at the NASA Goddard Space Flight Center in Greenbelt, Maryland during the 1980s. During his career as a network administrator, he resigned abruptly in 2006 due to an unknown debilitating health condition that was later learned to be Lyme disease.

You can follow *"The Lymester"* on YouTube for additional information or to contact the author.

30045078R00122

Made in the USA
San Bernardino, CA
21 March 2019